Living with Coronary Disease

D0829661

Clive Handler
Gerry Coghlan

Living with Coronary Disease

Foreword by Professor Dame Carol Black
DBE, FRCP, FMedSci

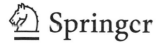 Springer

Clive Handler, BSc, MD, MRCP,
    FACC, FESC
Consultant Cardiologist
The National Pulmonary
    Hypertension Unit
The Royal Free Hospital
London, UK
and
Honorary Senior Lecturer
Department of Medicine
Royal Free and University
    College Medical School
London, UK
and
Consultant Cardiologist
Highgate Hospital
London, UK

Gerry Coghlan, MD, FRCP
Consultant Cardiologist
Department of Cardiology
The Royal Free Hospital
London, UK

British Library Cataloguing in Publication Data
A catalogue record for this book is available from the British Library

Library of Congress Control Number: 2006928328

ISBN-10: 1-84628-550-X   e-ISBN-10: 1-84628-551-8
ISBN-13: 978-1-84628-550-9   e-ISBN-13: 978-1-84628-551-6

9 8 7 6 5 4 3 2 1

Springer Science+Business Media
springer.com

Dr. Clive Handler dedicates this book to Caroline, Charlotte, Sophie, and Julius.

Dr. Coghlan dedicates this book to Eveleen, Niall, Cathal, and Eoin.

Foreword

Patients are increasingly and rightly demanding accessible and readily understandable information which enables them to be full partners in management decisions about their conditions. Organisations such as the British Heart Foundation and the American Heart Association have produced many helpful booklets explaining heart disease, and for many patients this is sufficient. However, for those who want self-help advice and a more comprehensive explanation of coronary artery disease, its cause, risk factors, how it is investigated, and its medical management, this book is an excellent companion.

"Living with Coronary Disease" uses terminology in every day use and each chapter can be read in isolation, giving the reader a thorough understanding of one particular aspect of the subject. The relationships between exercise, smoking, diet, and heart disease, are fully explained, and the reasons why not every smoker gets heart disease elucidated. "Living with Coronary Disease" helps you communicate with your doctor more effectively; it helps you understand why certain tests are necessary, what the results mean, when to rush to hospital and when not to worry too much.

This book meets the needs of anyone interested in understanding and avoiding coronary disease, and also helps those who have or know someone with heart problems, to live as normal a life as possible, avoiding future problems.

Professor Dame Carol Black DBE, FRCP, FMedSci
Chairman, Academy of Medical Royal Colleges, London
Emeritus Professor of Rheumatology
Royal Free Hospital, London

Preface

We are all more likely to die from a heart attack or a stroke than from any other condition including cancer or infections. Angina and heart attacks are due to narrowings and blockages in the heart arteries causing a lack of blood and oxygen to the heart. A stroke is due to lack of blood and oxygen to the brain. These heart and brain problems are due to stiffened and narrowed arteries due to deposits of fat called atheroma. This is more likely to occur if a person has certain risk factors. Fat in the heart arteries is called coronary heart disease and it is the commonest cause of death in the world.

Coronary heart disease affects men and women equally and starts in childhood. People of all ages, particularly the young, should understand what coronary heart disease is and what can be done to prevent it, or at least, delay it for as long as possible.

Although we do not fully understand how and why fat gets deposited in the arteries, we know that it is more likely to happen as we get older, in those who smoke, in those who have a high level of a fat called cholesterol or sugar (diabetes) in their blood, in those with high blood pressure (hypertension), and in those who are overweight and do little exercise. Stress is also bad for health and the heart but is more difficult to measure. These are called risk factors. Although many have been proposed, only a few account for the majority of problems. Coronary heart disease also runs in families although there is no single gene that accounts for this.

People without these risk factors are less likely to get angina, heart attacks, or strokes. People who have angina or have had a heart attack or a heart operation, improve their chances of a longer, more enjoyable life without further heart problems if they control and correct risk factors. This slows down the progression of fat deposition. The measures that really work are having a low blood level of cholesterol which is helped by eating very little fat – some people may need to take a tablet to lower the cholesterol – not smoking, making sure that the blood pressure is within the normal range, being slim and fit, and exercising frequently, preferably every day. These things are also very effective in reducing stress and make us feel better, stronger, more alert, and in better spirits.

A diagnosis of angina is made only if a person has symptoms of angina. The diagnosis is not made from a test. A diagnosis of a heart attack is made if a person has symptoms and an abnormal electrical recording of the heart (electrocardiogram, or ECG) and an abnormal blood test result. The treatment of angina and heart attacks has changed a lot in the last few years.

There is no doubt that if patients, their families, their doctors, and other clinicians involved in their care do their best and work together as a team, the outcome for patients will improve. The more people understand about this common condition, the more likely it is that they will be able to help themselves and reduce their risk of getting it in the first place. If they already have it, they will be able to improve their chances of living a longer, trouble-free life. Some things that have been proposed help a lot and others very little or not at all.

Both of us spend much of our working lives looking after patients with coronary heart disease. In order for patients and their families to receive the best care, they should understand their condition, what the tests and treatments involve – both the risks and the benefits – and which tests and treatments are the most appropriate for them. Although there are principles of treatment we can apply to all patients with angina and heart attacks, we try to tailor the tests and treatments to the patient because each case is different.

We have written this book for people who have coronary heart disease as well as for those who want to prevent it, including young people. We have tried to avoid medical jargon and have used simple, direct language in order to clarify a highly technical and complex subject.

We hope that you will enjoy this book and that it will dispel the natural fears of the condition and allow you to be more in control of your health and your future. It is important to remember that most people with coronary heart disease can and should lead a full, normal, and active life. If you look after your arteries and your heart, your heart will look after you.

Clive Handler
Gerry Coghlan
The Royal Free Hospital
London, UK

Acknowledgements

We would like to thank our patients and their families. Without them, we could not and would not have written this book. We would also like to thank our hospital colleagues and particularly the nurses, physiological technicians, and radiographers in our departments, who are very important members of the team. We are also grateful to our many colleagues in primary care, who help us care for our patients.

Dr. Clive Handler would like to thank his wife, Caroline, and his three children, Charlotte, Sophie, and Julius, for their support during the writing of this book. He would also like to thank Professor Lawrence Cohen MD, special adviser to the Dean, Yale University Medical School, who has emphasized the importance of clear communication with patients and their families.

The authors are also grateful to Charlotte Handler, Department of English, Bristol University, UK, and to Katie Wake, Department of History, University of Bristol, UK, for their help with editing the text, and to Dee Maclean for doing the illustrations.

Dr. Gerry Coghlan would like to thank his wife, Eveleen, and his three sons, Niall, Cathal, and Eoin, for their support during the writing of this book.

Contents

1

Angina and Heart Attacks: Overview

Read this chapter to learn about:

- coronary heart disease: what it is and the problems it causes
- angina
- heart attacks
- what makes angina and heart attacks more likely to occur and get worse (risk factors)
- what makes them less likely to occur.

We suggest you read this chapter first because it will give you an overview of the subject and so will make it easier to understand the rest of the book.

CORONARY HEART DISEASE IS THE MOST COMMON CAUSE OF DEATH IN THE WORLD

Cardiovascular disease is the main cause of death and disability in the developed world. Most men and women in developed countries will die from coronary heart disease rather than from cancer, AIDS, infections, or other diseases. Within a few years, it will also be biggest cause of death in young people.

The older we get, the more likely we are to get coronary heart disease. But there are things that we can all do to postpone it and reduce our chances of dying from it.

What Is Coronary Heart Disease?

It is a condition where a fatty substance (atheroma), consisting mainly of cholesterol, gets deposited on the inside lining of the walls of arteries. A chalky mineral (calcium) also gets deposited in the walls of the arteries as we age. These two processes cause the arteries to narrow and their walls become stiffer and less elastic. This is called atherosclerosis (athero = artery, sclerosis = hard) (figure 1.1).

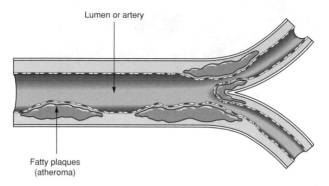

Lumen or artery

Fatty plaques
(atheroma)

Figure 1.1: Atherosclerosis: Plaques (layers) of fat (atheroma), mainly cholesterol, line the inside of arteries, initially outside the lumen, mainly in the heart, head, and neck arteries; the aorta; and the leg and kidney arteries. Atheroma does not occur in veins.

> *Coronary heart disease is fatty deposits in arteries and causes angina and heart attacks.*

WHAT CAUSES IT?

We do not know precisely how the fat gets into the walls of the arteries, but we do know that people with certain risk factors are more likely to get coronary heart disease than those who don't have those risk factors.

What Are Risk Factors?

Risk factors are conditions that make it more likely that a person will get a certain illness. Smoking is a risk factor for cancers, particularly lung cancer, as well as coronary heart disease. There are several other risk factors for coronary heart disease.

A person with a risk factor is more likely to get coronary heart disease compared to someone who does not have that risk factor. But just because a person has a risk factor, for example, being a smoker or having high cholesterol, does not mean that he will definitely get coronary heart disease. This explains why some people, albeit only a tiny minority, live to a good age, even if they smoke or have high cholesterol. Also, people without risk factors still get angina and die from a heart attack.

THE MORE RISK FACTORS A PERSON HAS, THE GREATER THEIR RISK

An overweight diabetic smoker who has high cholesterol and high blood pressure is many times more likely to get coronary heart disease than a person whose only risk factor is high blood pressure.

What Makes a Condition a Risk Factor?

It takes many years of observation and research to identify a risk factor. People had been smoking for several hundred years before it was proved that smoking was dangerous. It was only after it had been suggested that smoking could be a risk factor that studies could be done to test and prove this.

Whole communities of young people have to have their blood pressures, blood sugar levels, and cholesterol examined and tested , and then observed over many years to see if they get heart attacks or die earlier compared to those without these risk factors.

Recently, it has been reported that small babies who become overweight after the age of two years are more likely to die from heart attacks when they are adults than children who remain the correct weight for their age.

> *It is important for babies and young children to be given a healthy, low-fat, low-sugar, low-salt diet, as well as staying physically fit. They should also stay slim and not become overweight. If children get into good eating habits, they are less likely to die young from a heart attack.*

It has been known for 100 years that people who died from a heart attack had fat (cholesterol) in their arteries. Over the last 50 years, it has been confirmed that people with a lot of cholesterol in their blood are more likely to get angina and have a heart attack. The high cholesterol level is partly due to diet but there are other factors, for example, genetic factors, that are not fully understood.

For a Condition to be a Risk Factor, It Should

- at least double the risk of getting the disease
- apply to all people
- make scientific sense. It makes sense that a high level of cholesterol in the blood would lead to cholesterol deposits in arteries. It makes sense that high blood pressure would damage the walls of arteries
- removing the risk factor should lower the risk of getting the disease. This is why it is worthwhile for smokers to stop smoking, for obese people to lose weight, for people who do little or no exercise to exercise a lot, for people with high blood pressure or high cholesterol to take treatment to correct it, and for diabetics to control their blood sugar level

Things That Increase the Likelihood (Risk Factors) of a Person Getting Coronary Heart Disease (Furred Up Arteries)

These are now well established and accepted. They are

- getting older
- smoking
- high cholesterol (blood fat) level in the blood, particularly the "bad" LDL (low density lipoprotein) cholesterol
- high blood pressure (greater than 140/85)
- diabetes (high blood sugar level)
- being overweight
- stress
- not exercising regularly
- a family history of heart attack or angina below the age of 55 years of age.

It is thought that coronary heart disease occurs because several risk factors act together. It may be that some people are more vulnerable than others and get coronary heart disease at a younger age. Others may be less vulnerable to the same combination of risk factors.

> *The more risk factors a person has, the more likely he is to get coronary heart disease. For example, a person who smokes, is overweight, and has high blood pressure, diabetes and a high cholesterol level is at much greater risk of getting angina and a heart attack (as well as a stroke) than someone who has only one risk factor.*

> *A person can lower their risk of getting coronary heart disease if they "lose" or correct their risk factors. For example, a person who is overweight and who does no exercise, has a high sugar level, a high cholesterol level, and high blood pressure can "lose" five risk factors and greatly lower their risk of coronary heart disease, by losing weight and exercising. And it really works, too!*

WHAT CAN WE DO ABOUT RISK FACTORS?

Quite a lot. Some, like age and family history, cannot be modified. But we do have control over the others.

Some Risk Factors Are "Stronger" Than Others

Certain risk factors are stronger than others. A person who smokes 20 cigarettes per day is probably more likely to get coronary heart disease than someone whose only risk factor is being overweight.

A very high cholesterol level (particularly the "bad" LDL cholesterol) is a more potent risk factor than lack of exercise, or stress. A very high LDL cholesterol may be the most dangerous risk factor.

Graded Effect of Risk Factors

Some risk factors exert a "graded" effect. This applies to:

- the number of cigarettes smoked
- the amount of cholesterol in the blood
- blood pressure

The risk of developing coronary heart disease is related to, and increases with, the number of cigarettes smoked.

It may also apply to weight, but this has not been established.

Nearly all people with coronary heart disease have at least one risk factor.

We can't turn back the clock, but we are able to do quite a lot to help ourselves.

BUT SOME PEOPLE GET CORONARY HEART DISEASE AND HAVE NO RISK FACTORS!

True, but not many. Coronary heart disease is very uncommon in people who have *no* risk factors. The risk factors listed above account for the vast majority of cases of coronary heart disease. Smokers often know of someone who "smoked all his life and lived to a ripe old age!" Maybe so, but he (or she) may have had a bad chest with bronchitis and emphysema and may have died from his lung problems or cancer of the lung or another part of the body, before dying from a heart attack. Most smokers know that if they continue, it will catch up with them sooner than they would like.

Things That Lower the Risk of Coronary Heart Disease

- Young age
- Never having smoked or having stopped completely more than 10 years ago. Someone who stopped smoking more than 10 years previously has the same risk of getting coronary heart disease as someone who has never smoked. The risk of getting coronary heart disease is reduced the first day that a smoker stops smoking. The sooner smokers stop, the sooner they lower their risk
- Normal blood pressure (less than 140/85)
- Low cholesterol level (LDL cholesterol less than 2.0 mmol/l)
- High "good" HDL cholesterol level
- Low-fat, healthy diet (fresh fruit and vegetables). Avoiding junk food
- Doing lots of exercise (30 minutes of hard, sweaty cardiovascular exercise per day – running, jogging, cycling are best)
- Being slim (flat tummy)

- Having a normal blood sugar level – no diabetes
- Low-stress levels, relaxed, chilled out as much of the time as possible, content, at ease and in control
- Having fit, healthy parents in their 90s (this is not so easy to arrange!)
- One unit of alcohol per day (remember all alcohol is fattening, particularly, beer).

WHAT IS LIFESTYLE?

It's the way we live our lives and the effects it has on our mental and physical health.

Where we live; who we live with; whether we live alone or with a spouse or partner; our job; where we work; how we get to work or whether we work from home; whether we like our job and the people we work with and whether we are fulfilled and happy; how much time we have to do the things we want to do; our responsibilities to our family, our children, our friends; whether we spend our lives doing something we enjoy most of the time or something we find oppressive, boring, depressing, and stressful; what and how much we eat, when we eat; how much alcohol we drink; the stresses we are under (both self-induced and those out of our control); if we smoke or take drugs; how much useful exercise we do; our enjoyment of sex; how much good-quality sleep we get; our mood, our spirits and our feeling of satisfaction with ourselves and contentment with "our lot," whether we are able to laugh at a joke, make a joke and enjoy ourselves; our relationships with the people we live and work with, our ambitions and how we feel about ourselves and what we think other people think of us.

Lifestyle is everything connected to, or underlying, the way we spend every hour of the day.

COUNTING OUR BLESSINGS AND BEING GRATEFUL FOR THE GOOD THINGS

Every aspect of our life is a potential source of both enjoyment and stress. There may be things we take for granted that give us pleasure, pride, and contentment. One of the helpful ways to

---

deal with stress is to remind ourselves of the good things in our lives and be grateful for these.

IS THERE A GENE FOR CORONARY HEART DISEASE?

No. A gene for coronary heart disease has not so far been discovered. This may mean that coronary heart disease does not occur for one simple reason but is the result of lots of different things, acting together.

Coronary heart disease does run in families. This may be because they have a high cholesterol level. A gene for high cholesterol has been found and this can be passed on.

GOOD HABITS SHOULD START BEFORE BIRTH

Fat is deposited in the walls of arteries at a young age in some people and is present in some children. Layers of fat have also been found in stillbirths of mothers who have smoked and have had a bad diet during pregnancy. This is why it is so important for pregnant women to be careful and protect their baby, not only from the effects of smoking, drugs, alcohol, and nearly all medications, but also from the effects of an unhealthy, high-fat, high-salt diet.

They should remember that the fat in their blood circulates to their baby. Fat babies often become fat children and fat adults. Fat adults are more likely to get coronary heart disease.

IMPORTANCE OF PREVENTION OF CORONARY HEART DISEASE IN CHILDHOOD

Children should be educated about health matters by example at home and in school. This means that parents can do a lot to guide and educate their children. If parents smoke, drink too much alcohol or have a bad diet, their children are likely to inherit these habits and thus have a higher risk of getting coronary heart disease at a needlessly young age.

Children whose parents are fit, slim, eat a healthy diet, don't smoke, don't drink excessively, and exercise regularly are less likely to get coronary heart disease than children whose parents have an unhealthy lifestyle.

ARE WE ALL GOING TO GET CORONARY HEART DISEASE?

Probably yes, if we live long enough because it is part of aging. However, it may not be the main reason we die. A person may have coronary heart disease but die of a chest infection or kidney failure rather than a heart attack.

Does It Affect Men More Than Women?

No. It affects men and women equally, although it affects women at an older age. Coronary heart disease is not a male disease. For many years it was thought to affect men more than women. This is no longer the case.

But Aren't Women More Likely to Die From Breast Cancer?

No. Women are more likely to die from a heart attack than cancer of the breast or cancer of the womb. This may be due to their changing role in society: more women smoke than they used to and they also work longer hours and in more stressful jobs than they did 50 years ago. With their traditional home-making and mothering roles, many are juggling three busy jobs, which places high demands on their time. Women become vulnerable to coronary heart disease after menopause (see figure 1.1).

WHY DOES FAT IN A HEART ARTERY CAUSE SO MUCH TROUBLE?

- Narrowing of the heart arteries and reduced flow of blood and oxygen to the heart, causing angina (figure 1.2)

The fat in the artery restricts the flow of blood and oxygen to the heart muscle. This may provoke a symptom called *angina*.

- Cracking of the surface of the layer of fat, formation of a blood clot blocking the artery, causing a *heart attack*

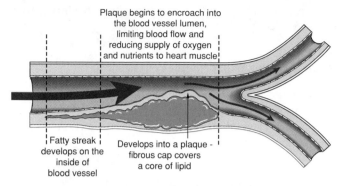

Plaque begins to encroach into the blood vessel lumen, limiting blood flow and reducing supply of oxygen and nutrients to heart muscle

Fatty streak develops on the inside of blood vessel

Develops into a plaque - fibrous cap covers a core of lipid

Figure 1.2: Stages of atherosclerosis: as the plaque gets bigger, it begins to block off the artery. If more than 70% of the width of an artery is blocked or narrowed, the flow of blood and oxygen is reduced. In the heart arteries, this may cause angina.

The plaque is covered by a cap of cells. If the fat is hard and "stable," it may be safe and not "crack," or rupture. A ruptured cap of cells over a plaque containing soft fat can cause a heart attack or unstable angina.

For reasons that are not clear, the top surface of the fat layer (plaque) may crack. A blood clot forms on top of the plaque, and if big enough, may block off the artery completely. This blocks the supply of blood and oxygen to the heart muscle, causing a heart attack and death of part of the heart muscle (*myocardial infarction*), which is often fatal. This usually happens suddenly and can also occur without warning (figure 1.3).

THE FINANCIAL, SOCIAL, AND PSYCHOLOGICAL COSTS OF CORONARY HEART DISEASE

Coronary heart disease is one of the most common cause of death in the world and is becoming increasingly widespread as life expectancy increases. It consumes a lot of a country's economy due to lost income and health benefits when young people can no longer work; the costs of treatment – medicines and operations – are expensive.

People of all ages die from a heart attack. Older people are more likely to die than younger people. Younger people

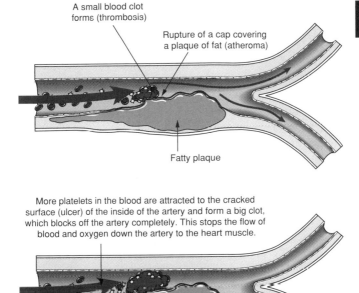

A small blood clot forms (thrombosis)

Rupture of a cap covering a plaque of fat (atheroma)

Fatty plaque

More platelets in the blood are attracted to the cracked surface (ulcer) of the inside of the artery and form a big clot, which blocks off the artery completely. This stops the flow of blood and oxygen down the artery to the heart muscle.

Figure 1.3: The cause of heart attacks, unstable angina, and death: Rupture of a plaque and clot, causing blockage of an artery with blood clot (platelet cells) and heart attack.

are more likely to be able to return to work and live a normal life after a heart attack.

Many more people of working age may survive a heart attack, but are left with a weakened heart muscle (heart failure), which may make it difficult for them to continue working. This affects their families, friends, and their businesses. Many of those who survive cannot work again due to physical and emotional disability.

Coronary heart disease causes depression, lack of confidence, and stress within a family. This is a big problem, and there is growing interest in ways to tackle this with cardiac rehabilitation programmes.

WHAT PROBLEMS CAN CORONARY HEART DISEASE CAUSE?

It can cause several:

- of those dying before reaching hospital, 70% die suddenly from a leathal heart rhythm abnormality (ventricular fibrillation)
- disability following a heart attack and increased risk of another heart attack
- weakening of the heart (heart failure) causing breathlessness, fatigue, exhaustion, leg swelling
- angina
- heart rhythm abnormalities leading to palpitations, dizziness, and loss of consciousness
- anxiety, depression, stress, and loss of confidence
- loss of libido, impotence and an unhappy, strained personal relationship.

WHAT DO THE WORDS "CORONARY HEART DISEASE" MEAN?

The word "coronary" refers to a problem with a **heart artery** rather than another part of the heart. All other parts of the heart can be affected by other types of disease.

The heart artery gets narrowed due to a buildup of fat (cholesterol) mixed with blood cells and calcium in the inside of the arteries of the heart. This condition is often likened to furring up and narrowing of a water pipe because there is slower flow of blood in the artery (figure 1.1).

Arteries are the tubes (blood vessels) that carry blood-containing oxygen and nutrients to all the organs of the body. We cannot live without oxygen. If the oxygen supply is reduced to any part of the body, problems occur.

The two main problems resulting from coronary heart disease are angina and heart attack.

- Angina – what causes it and what does it feel like?
  If the heart muscle is deprived of blood and oxygen it cannot pump and perform its job properly. This causes chest tightness, heaviness, discomfort or breathlessness. These symptoms may spread to the arms, neck, back or stomach. It usually occurs during exercise (particularly after a heavy

meal) or stress, or in cold weather, lasts for a few minutes, and passes off within a few minutes with rest.

HOW DOES A DOCTOR KNOW THAT A PERSON HAS ANGINA?

A diagnosis of angina is made from what the patient tells us; not by a test. That is why it is so important for patients to describe what they feel but also for the doctor to listen very carefully to what patients tell them.

> *Patients with angina should see their GP, who may refer them to a cardiologist (a consultant specialising in heart problems) for tests and further treatment.*

- Heart attack – what causes it and what does it feel like?
  If the blood supply to the heart muscle is cut off for more than 30 minutes, this may damage, scar, and weaken the area of heart muscle supplied by the blocked artery. The cells of the heart muscle die because they cannot live without oxygen and nutrients. Death of heart muscle cells is called a heart attack (myocardial infarct).
  A heart attack is diagnosed from the patient's description of what he felt, by a blood test, and by an electrical recording of the heart (ECG).

WHAT DOES A HEART ATTACK FEEL LIKE?

Sudden, severe, central or left-sided chest pain. This is commonly described as pressure, squeezing, breathlessness with sweating, and sometimes sickness and vomiting. Some people pass out. Some people feel "as if an elephant is sitting on their chest". The symptoms last at least 20 minutes and the pain in the chest may also be felt in the throat, jaws, and arms.

Although there are several conditions that can mimic angina, there are fewer things that mimic a heart attack. Some of these are equally dangerous and need to be investigated urgently.

> *People with a suspected heart attack should dial for an emergency ambulance and the paramedics and go to the hospital for tests and treatment.*

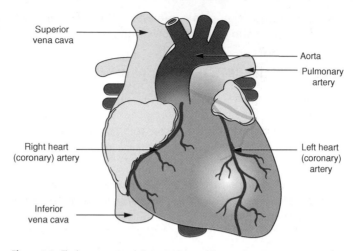

Figure 1.4: The heart – external view.

APART FROM CORONARY HEART DISEASE, WHAT ARE THE OTHER TYPES OF HEART DISEASE?

Apart from a problem with the arteries, there are other types of heart disease depending on which part of the heart is affected.

Apart from the two main heart arteries (one on the left called the left coronary artery and one on the right called the right coronary artery), which are on the surface of the heart muscle, the heart consists of

- four valves
- muscle
- a membrane covering the heart called the pericardium (peri = around, cardium = the heart).

IF WE DON'T DIE FROM A HEART ATTACK OR A STROKE, WHAT ARE WE LIKELY TO DIE FROM?

Not all old people die from coronary heart disease. Many die from "old age"; worn-out kidneys, dementia, an infection (for example, a bad chest infection or pneumonia) or cancer. Cancer is not as common a cause of death as heart attacks, heart failure, and stroke. Elderly people who develop cancer frequently

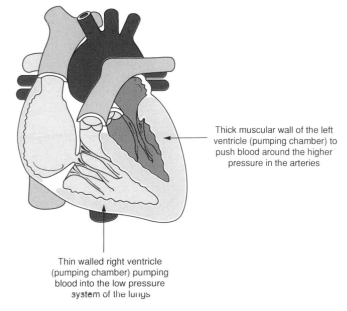

Thick muscular wall of the left ventricle (pumping chamber) to push blood around the higher pressure in the arteries

Thin walled right ventricle (pumping chamber) pumping blood into the low pressure system of the lungs

Figure 1.5: The heart – internal view: The heart opened up from the front.

die from cardiovascular disease rather than their cancer because many forms of cancer grow slowly in the elderly.

We should not forget that in some developing countries, malaria, AIDS, childhood infections, starvation, famine, and drought are responsible for the deaths of lots of people.

WE ARE LIVING LONGER WITH CORONARY HEART DISEASE AND AFTER HEART ATTACKS. WHY?

Because medical care and treatment have improved. We understand more about how these conditions develop and how we can reduce our risk of getting coronary heart disease.

- Quitting smoking
  Fewer adults smoke due to anti-smoking publicity, smoking clinics, help-lines and medications (although smoking among children, teenagers, and the 20-year-olds, particularly females, may be increasing). It is also likely that fewer people will smoke

and be affected by passive smoking when smoking is banned in public places.

- Diet
  Most people accept that they will live longer if they are slim, active and have a good, low-fat, low-salt, low-sugar diet.
- Drugs
  The medications we prescribe for patients with coronary heart disease – aspirin (which reduces the stickiness of the blood), beta blockers (which lower the blood pressure and the heart rate), statins (which lower the cholesterol level but have other useful effects, too), drugs that work on the kidneys and are good for the heart and the arteries (angiotensin converting enzyme inhibitors or ACE inhibitors) – are the drugs that, together, have made a big impact in prolonging life in patients who have coronary heart disease.
- Exercise and weight
  Healthy eating and exercise are beneficial. Thinner people live longer and are more likely to survive longer after a heart attack.
- High blood pressure, high cholesterol level, and diabetes
  High blood pressure, and high cholesterol levels and diabetes, are treated better and more aggressively in everyone, particularly those with coronary heart disease. These measures are helpful in slowing the progress of coronary heart disease.
- Identifying people at high risk
  This is difficult, but there are tests that can show which people are at high risk of having a heart attack. People who can exercise on a treadmill or cycle for at least 10 minutes, without getting angina, or becoming unduly breathless, and whose blood pressure increases normally, and who do not get abnormal changes in the electrical recording of their heart, or abnormal heart rhythms during the exercise (stress) test, are at relatively low risk for further problems after a heart attack. However, these "low-risk" individuals also need to adopt a healthy lifestyle.

Cholesterol Gets Deposited in Arteries Other Than the Heart Arteries – Cardiovascular Disease

Although this book deals with coronary heart disease causing angina and heart attacks, it is important to remember that cholesterol gets deposited in other arteries, too, causing other common problems.

Cardiovascular (cardio = heart, vascular = blood vessel) disease (or simply, vascular disease) is the term used to describe cholesterol or atheroma affecting not only the heart (coronary) arteries, but also arteries supplying the brain, the neck, the kidneys and the legs. Why these arteries are affected more commonly than other arteries in the body is not clear. Blockages in the blood supply to these parts of the body have important consequences.

Cardiovascular Disease: Effects of Fatty Deposits in Arteries Other Than the Heart Arteries

Cholesterol deposits affect

- The brain arteries (*cerebrovascular disease*) causing *strokes*. A stroke may cause weakness of one side of the body and loss of, or difficulty with, speech.
- The kidney arteries (*renovascular disease*), causing *kidney failure and high blood pressure.*
- The leg arteries (*peripheral vascular disease*), causing leg cramps and *pain in the legs and buttocks when walking (claudication).*
- The aorta (the main blood vessel carrying blood out from the heart), causing narrowing and reduced blood supply to the legs. If a person also has a high blood pressure, the wall of the aorta can tear (dissect), get weak, and there may be a blow out (aneurysm). A rupture is usually fatal.
- The blood supply to the penis causing impotence. It is now well established that impotence (erectile dysfunction) may be an early sign of vascular disease. Therefore, men with impotence should be examined and tested for coronary heart disease or other forms of vascular disease. Men with coronary heart disease should bear in mind that if they have angina and impotence, the two conditions may be connected.

DOES CHOLESTEROL GET INTO THE VEINS?

No, Cholesterol does not get deposited in veins (the blood vessels carrying blood back to the heart from all parts of the body).

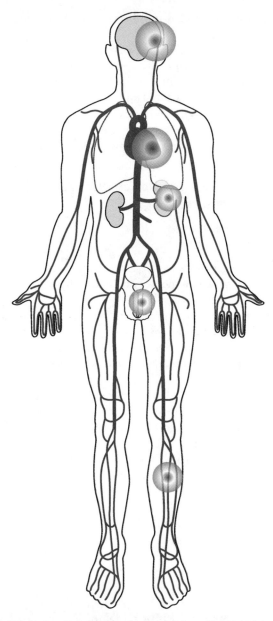

Figure 1.6: Systemic problems: Common sites where cholesterol is deposited. Atherosclerosis, due to cholesterol deposits, affects the arteries supplying blood to the heart, the brain, the kidneys, the penis, and the leg arteries.

This is because the pressure in veins is very much lower than in arteries.

How cholesterol gets into the wall of arteries is not clear, but it may have something to do with the pressure inside the artery forcing the cholesterol circulating in the blood, into the arterial wall. If the pressure in an artery is higher than it should be (hypertension), then it is more likely that cholesterol will be forced into the wall of the artery.

CAN WE GET RID OF CORONARY HEART DISEASE?

No. Once fat has been deposited inside an artery it cannot be re-moved completely. Modern treatments, such as the cholesterol-lowering drugs called statins, combined with a low-fat diet and vigorous daily exercise, may help reduce the amount of fat inside the artery. Statins (which can now be bought, like aspirin, "over the counter") reduce the cholesterol level, reduce the inflam-mation in the arteries, and convert a lump of soft, inflamed fat which is likely to crack (an unstable fatty plaque) into a sta-ble plaque. So even though there may be fat in an artery, it can be changed into a relatively harmless type of fat. This reduces the risk of heart attacks and can improve symptoms of angina. We now give statins to everyone who has had a heart attack and has coronary or any other form of vascular disease.

2

The Heart: How It Works and What Can Go Wrong

In this chapter we explain:

- what the heart is
- the heart's structure and component parts
- how the heart works
- how blood circulates in the body
- what can happen when the heart doesn't work properly.

THE HEART AND THE CIRCULATION

The heart consists of two pumps joined side to side. There are two parallel circulations.

Stale blood with has had oxygen removed by all the organs of the body, travels in veins back to the right side of the heart. It is then pumped by the right side of the heart to the lungs, where it picks up oxygen from the air we breathe.

The fresh blood containing oxygen then travels to the left side of the heart.

The blood, which has been oxygenated in the lungs, is then pumped around the body by the left heart pump (the left ventricle). The blood is carried in arteries to supply all the cells in all the organs and body parts, enabling them to perform their functions (figure 2.1).

The phase when the heart squeezes blood out is called *systole*. The phase when the heart fills with blood is called *diastole* (figure 2.2).

Blood pressure is measured and recorded using both of these phases. So a recording of 120/80, measured in mm of mercury (Hg), is a pressure of 120 in the arteries when the heart is squeezing (systole or systolic blood pressure), and 80 (diastolic blood pressure) when the heart is relaxing and filling with blood.

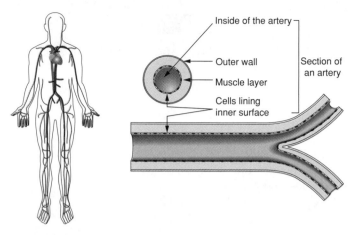

Inside of the artery

Outer wall

Muscle layer

Cells lining
inner surface

Section of
an artery

The heart and the main
arteries of the body

Figure 2.1: Arteries and circulation: Arteries, compared to veins, have thick, muscular walls to withstand high blood pressure. Veins have thin walls, and the pressure inside is much lower.

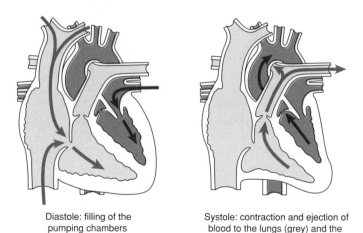

Diastole: filling of the
pumping chambers

Systole: contraction and ejection of
blood to the lungs (grey) and the
rest of the body (red)

Figure 2.2: Diastole/systole.

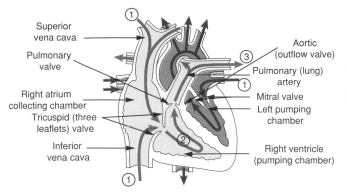

Figure 2.3: Blood flow through heart: Grey (1) blood enters the right collecting chamber (atrium) from the upper body through the superior vena cava, and from the lower body through the inferior vena cava. It then passes through the tricuspid value, between the right atrium and right ventricle, into the right ventricle (2) and then through the pulmonary valve into the pulmonary (lung) artery (3). It is then pushed into the arteries of both lungs where it picks up oxyzen. Red: (1) Blood, rich in oxygen, having passed through the lungs, enters the left atrium (collecting chamber). It then passes through the mitral valve and then into the muscular left ventricle (2). It is then squeezed into the main blood vessel, the aorta, through the aortic valve. (NB: Filling of both atria occurs simultaneously and contraction or squeezing of both ventricles occurs simultaneously.)

WHAT DOES "CIRCULATION" MEAN?

Circulation means the flow of blood around the body.

WHAT DOES THE HEART LOOK LIKE?

The heart is a hard-working pump made of dark red muscle the size of an adult fist. It is shaped like a blunt-ended cone.

Where is the heart?

The heart is found just beneath and to the left of the breastbone (sternum). When we lean forward or lie on our left side, the heart falls against the rib cage, which is why people often feel their heartbeat (palpitation) when lying in bed. If you can't feel it, it does not mean your heart is not beating! The heartbeat is less easily felt in people with a thick chest wall or if they have emphysema (lots of air in the lung airspaces).

The structure of the heart (see figure 1.4)

The heart consists of

- two pumps joined side by side but separated by a thin partition wall called the *septum*
- four hollow chambers. The two pumping chambers are called *ventricles*. The two collecting or receiving chambers are called *atria*
- four valves, which control the flow and direction of blood around the heart. There are two on the left and two on the right side of the heart (see figure 1.5).

The left side of the heart

The left side of the heart consists of

- the left collecting chamber (*left atrium*), which receives fresh blood containing oxygen from the lungs.
- the *mitral valve*, which is situated between the left atrium and the left ventricle. When open, it allows blood to flow from the left atrium to the left ventricle. When closed, it prevents blood from leaking back from the ventricle to the atrium.
- the left pumping chamber (*left ventricle*), which pumps blood around the body. It is much thicker than the right ventricle because it has to pump blood against a higher pressure and therefore has more work to do.
- the *aortic valve,* which is situated between the left ventricle and the main arterial trunk called the *aorta*. When open, it allows blood to be ejected from the ventricle into the aorta for distribution around the body. When closed, it prevents ejected blood from leaking back from the aorta into the ventricle.

The right side of the heart

The right heart side of the heart consists of

- the right collecting chamber (*right atrium*), which receives stale blood containing very little oxygen
- the *tricuspid valve,* which is situated between the right atrium and the right ventricle. When open, it allows blood flow from

---

the right atrium to the right ventricle. When closed, it prevents blood from leaking back from the ventricle to the atrium

- the right pumping chamber (*right ventricle*), which pumps blood to the lungs for refreshment with oxygen. It pumps blood into a low-pressure system in the lungs, and its walls are thinner than those of the left ventricle because it has less work to do

- the *pulmonary valve*, which is situated between the right ventricle and the main artery to the lungs (*pulmonary artery*). When open, it allows blood to be ejected from the ventricle into the pulmonary artery for distribution around the lung arteries, arterioles (smaller lung arteries) and capillaries. When closed, it prevents blood from leaking back from the pulmonary artery into the ventricle.

What Can Go Wrong with the Left Side of the Heart?

Apart from the coronary arteries, problems can develop in each part of the heart.

Valve problems

There are several types of valve problems. Four valves control the flow of blood through the heart. There are two on the right side of the heart and two on the left side.

Blood should flow forward through the heart. The valves may get narrowed or leaky or, both narrowed and leaky. If the valves do not work properly, this may damage the heart muscle and lead to weakness of the heart. Various conditions may affect the valves.

Infections (for example, *rheumatic fever*) may damage any of the four heart valves although the valves in the left side of the heart (the mitral and aortic) are the ones most commonly affected. The valves on the left side of the heart may be damaged over time for the same reasons that heart arteries get narrowed. The valve tissue and the area of the heart muscle in which they are situated may get affected by chalky deposits of calcium (see figure 2.3).

Aortic valve problems
A narrow aortic valve – aortic stenosis.   As we get older, and also for the same reasons that arteries get furred up (blocked with

fatty deposits), the aortic outflow valve may get thickened, worn out, and not open fully. This is called *aortic stenosis*.

If the valve narrows, the left ventricle has to work harder to squeeze blood through a smaller outlet and against a higher pressure. The only way it can do this is for the walls to get thicker. High blood pressure is a common cause of a thickened heart muscle for the same reason.

Problems due to a narrowed aortic valve

- *Angina*. The thickened heart muscle needs more oxygen, in the same way as a big engine needs more gas.
- *Fainting or loss of consciousness* (*syncope*) may occur if the valve opening gets so narrow that not enough blood gets out of the heart to the head. This most commonly occurs during exercise when the blood is diverted to the muscles of the legs and arms, decreasing the amount available for the head and brain.
- *Breathlessness*. After many years of working hard, pumping blood against a high pressure, the left ventricle thickens, enlarges, and then fails, causing *heart failure*. By this time, it may be too late for the patient to benefit from a new valve. It is important for aortic stenosis to be diagnosed before the heart fails so that the old valve can be replaced.

A leaky aortic valve – *aortic regurgitation.* This is less common than a narrowed aortic valve. The valve does not close properly and blood leaks back into the ventricle, putting a strain on the heart. The causes include old age, high blood pressure, infections on the valve due to rheumatic fever or endocarditis and rarely, some arthritic conditions (but not osteoarthritis).

Both a narrowed and leaky aortic valve are diagnosed with heart ultrasound (echocardiography). If the valve is severely narrowed, it may need replacing.

Mitral valve problems

A narrowed mitral valve – *mitral stenosis.* This is caused by rheumatic fever in childhood, but the valve becomes narrow only several years later. Rheumatic fever is more common in less economically developed countries. It is now comparatively rare in the UK and the US.

The narrowed mitral valve obstructs blood flow from the left atrium into the left ventricle. The pressure increases in the left atrium, which gets bigger. The increased pressure is transmitted back through the lungs. Fluid accumulates in the lungs causing breathlessness (*pulmonary edema*). The water in the lung air sacs interferes with the transfer of oxygen getting into the bloodstream from the air we breathe. In very severe cases, the high pressure in the lungs is transmitted to the pulmonary arteries and back to the right side of the heart, causing failure of the right heart.

A narrowed mitral valve can be diagnosed with heart ultrasound (echocardiogram). It can be treated by stretching and widening the mitral valve using a special balloon (mitral valvuloplasty) inserted from the groin, or with an operation (mitral valvotomy). If the valve is both leaky and narrowed, it may be necessary to replace the valve.

Causes of a leaky mitral valve

- Floppy mitral valve – *mitral valve prolapse*. Quite commonly, in around 10% of people (typically young, tall, slim females), the mitral valve may be malformed and the segments of the valve are too big. In over 90% of people this does not cause a problem. However, a very leaky mitral valve can become problematic. Very occasionally, the very thin and delicate muscle strings that control the opening and closing of the mitral valve (like the cords on a parachute) break, resulting suddenly in a torrent of blood flooding back into the left atrium (mitral regurgitation) and into the lungs (pulmonary edema). This causes sudden breathlessness and a sensation of drowning. Urgent heart surgery is required to mend the valve.
- *Mitral regurgitation.* The mitral valve may also become leaky if the tiny muscles that control the muscle strings are damaged by a heart attack.

The mitral valve may become both narrowed and leaky several years after an attack of rheumatic fever in childhood. They are most commonly affected if the pressure is high in the lungs (pulmonary arterial hypertension).

Problems with the Tricuspid Valve in the Right Side of the Heart

The *tricuspid valve* (the inflow valve regulating blood flow from the right collecting chamber to the right pumping chamber) is less commonly affected than the valves on the left side of the heart. It is most commonly affected if the right pumping chamber has to pump against high pressure in the lungs. This is called *pulmonary hypertension*. The common causes of this are bronchitis and emphysema caused by smoking. The right ventricle is not as strong or powerful as the left pumping chamber and so it stretches and enlarges if it has to pump against a high pressure. If the chambers stretch, the valve is stretched and may leak because the valve segments are pulled apart.

Pulmonary hypertension

The most common cause is damage to the lungs from smoking. The smoke destroys the capillaries and the very small airspaces in the lungs, increasing the pressure in the main arteries. There are other very rare causes of high pressure in the lung arteries.

Any cause of high pressure in the lungs will put a strain on the right pumping chamber, which stretches and weakens. This in turn stretches the tricuspid valve, which is situated between the right atrium and the right ventricle. The stretched valve may become leaky, allowing blood to leak back from the right ventricle to the right atrium.

Infective endocarditis

This is an uncommon and dangerous condition. This condition does not affect people with a normal heart.

It is due to an infection in the bloodstream traveling to the heart and damaging the valves. The bugs travel in the blood and land on a faulty heart valve or a hole in the heart, settle, multiply, and damage the valve.

It can affect any valve but most commonly affects the tricuspid valve in drug addicts who inject themselves with dirty drugs, through infected skin and using dirty needles. However careful they may be, repeated injections (mainlining) are a common cause of this dangerous infection.

This infection can also infect faulty valves on the left side of the heart following dental treatment or certain procedures, for example, instruments inserted in people with bowel or urinary problems. Bugs from the mouth (and we all have them), get into the bloodstream during certain types of dental work, for example, digging around gums.

This infection is difficult to treat. If patients with a heart valve problem feel tired, sweaty or experience appetite and or weight loss, they should see their doctor for tests and they may need to go into hospital. Infective endocarditis is a potentially fatal condition and is treated in hospital with a six-week course of antibiotics given into the veins. If the heart valve is damaged by the infection or the infection cannot be cured with antibiotics, it will need to be replaced, but this is a risky operation.

Preventing infective endocarditis

People with a heart valve problem or a hole in the heart are advised to take an antibiotic before any procedure that could lead to infection in the bloodstream. The GP will give the prescription depending on what procedure is to be done and whether the patient has any allergies to certain antibiotics.

Antibiotics are not necessary for people with coronary heart disease or who have had ballooning of their heart arteries (angioplasty) or heart bypass surgery, unless they have an abnormal valve.

What is a heart murmur?

A *murmur* is a sound heard with a stethoscope. It is due to flow of blood through the heart. Heart murmurs may occur in a normal person or be sign of a problem with an abnormal heart valve or a hole in the heart.

Murmurs in a normal heart

It is possible to hear blood flowing through the heart in *normal people*, particularly in children, and in young or slim people with a thin chest wall. This is because their heart is not far beneath the surface of the skin and so it is often easy to hear the flow of blood. People with a normal heart may have a heart murmur if the flow of blood in their heart is fast. This commonly occurs after exercise, if they are nervous (for example, being examined), and during pregnancy when the amount of blood in the circulation is increased due to the added circulation of the baby.

Murmurs in an abnormal heart

Abnormal heart murmurs are due to abnormal flow in the heart and turbulence. This can be due to a heart valve abnormality (narrowed, leaky or both narrow and leaky), a hole in the heart (or other problem that a person is born with – a congenital problem), or due to a very vigorous, strong heart with thickened walls.

Heart murmurs are louder on the left side of the heart because the pressure is higher compared to the right side. Heart murmurs are not painful. If a valve is very narrowed or leaky, it puts a strain on the heart muscle and this, over time, can cause heart failure. Patients who have been told that they have a heart murmur should ask their doctor if it is due to a faulty valve or other structural problem and if they need antibiotics before procedures or operations that could spread infection into the blood, damaging the valve.

Heart Ultrasound – Echocardiography

Ultrasound of the heart (echocardiography) is harmless and the best way to see if a murmur is due to an abnormal heart valve or other structural problem, or if it is normal and nothing to worry about.

Heart muscle disease

If the heart pump is weak, this causes heart failure. This can be mild or severe and the symptoms depend on how bad it is.

Symptoms of heart failure

- shortness of breath
- tiredness
- swollen ankles and feet
- dry cough
- loss of appetite, constipation, and bloating of the tummy.

Causes of heart failure

- Weakening of the heart due to *untreated or uncontrolled high blood pressure* and damage after a heart attack are the most common causes.
  High blood pressure (*hypertension*) puts the heart under pressure because it has to force blood around the circulation. The walls of the heart thicken in order to generate a higher pumping pressure, but eventually, if the blood pressure is not controlled

at a lower level, the heart muscle enlarges and fails. This is the main reason for checking and treating high blood pressure.

- *Valve problems.* If the heart loses its shape because it has enlarged or the walls are thicker, it gets weaker. A leaky or narrowed heart valve may also cause heart failure and this is the main reason that heart valves are replaced and, in some cases, repaired.
- *Heart attacks* are an increasingly common cause of heart failure. This is because more people are surviving heart attacks, living longer but with a weakened heart muscle.
- Heart failure is common in people who are *overweight and obese* because the excess weight puts a strain on the heart. They are more likely to get coronary heart disease and get heart attacks.
- People who smoke may get *bronchitis and emphysema* of their lungs. These conditions affect the blood pressure in the lung arteries, and this may put a strain on the right side of the heart (which is responsible for pumping blood into the lungs for oxygen enrichment). If the right side of the heart fails, this can cause swelling of the legs and breathlessness.
- Less commonly, there may be a problem with the heart muscle – *cardiomyopathy* (cardio = heart, myo — muscle, and pathy = abnormal). There are a number of different types of cardiomyopathy. They may all cause a weakening of the heart.
  If the *heart muscle is thickened* and stiff, we call this *hypertrophic cardiomyopathy* (hypertrophy = thickened). This is less common than high blood pressure as a cause of a thickened heart muscle. It has been found to be the cause of deaths in young athletes. Some forms are due to a genetic problem and so the close relatives of patients should be checked. The heart muscle may also get thick in people who do a lot of exercise (athlete's heart).

When the *heart is enlarged and saggy*, we call this *dilated cardiomyopathy*. This type can be caused by excess alcohol consumption.

Pericardial Disease

The membrane lining around the heart (*pericardium*) may get infected or inflamed and scarred (*pericarditis* = inflammation of the lining around the heart). This can cause chest pain, fever and a flu-like illness.

Pericardial problems are unusual. There are several ways to investigate them using heart ultrasound (echocardiogram) and new methods of imaging. These include computerised tomography (CT scanning) and magnetic resonance imaging.

WHAT IS BLOOD PRESSURE?

Blood would not move and circulate around the body unless it was pushed around by the heart pump. The pressure in the arteries depends on:

- the power of the heart pump. If the pump is weak, the pressure may be low.
- the volume of blood in the circulation. If there is little blood in the circulation, for example after loss of a lot of blood, the pressure may be low.
- the resistance against which the heart has to pump. This depends on the diameter of the smaller arteries called arterioles. If the arterioles are narrowed, the pressure is high. If the arterioles are relaxed and wide open, the pressure is low. Arteries have muscular walls and can expand and narrow down quickly when necessary to maintain the blood pressure if it is low.

One of the main reasons for high blood pressure is the arterioles are clamped down, increasing the blood pressure. Why they clamp down is not known, but several of the drugs used to treat high blood pressure widen the arteries (vasodilators, vaso = vessel, dilator = to open).

Blood pressure is measured in millimeters of mercury because that is how it was measured many years ago. The abbreviation is mm Hg.

What is High Blood Pressure?

High blood pressure is a blood pressure consistently above 140/85. The higher the blood pressure, the greater the risk of stroke, heart attacks and all types of arterial disease.

What Is the Pulse?

The pulse we feel at the wrist is the force of the wave of blood pumped out of the left heart. A pulse can be felt anywhere in the body where an artery lies just under the skin:

- at the front of the elbow (brachial artery)
- in the groin at the top of each leg (femoral artery)
- at the front of the foot in line with the big toe (foot artery)
- in front of each ear (temporal artery)
- behind each knee (popliteal artery).

What is an artery?

Arteries are blood vessels that carry fresh, bright red blood containing oxygen and nutrients around the body. Arteries have thick, elastic, muscular walls to withstand the high pressure pumped by the heart. The pressure in the arteries is called the blood pressure and should be at or below 140/85 mmHg (it is measured in mm of mercury). The walls of arteries may get harder and narrowed with fat (atherosclerosis) under certain conditions (see right hand panel of figure 2.1).

The main arterial trunk: The aorta

The main artery that starts at the outflow of the left side of the heart and is the main artery carrying fresh blood around the body is called the *aorta*. It is around one inch in diameter and extends from the heart, upward toward the neck and then down through the chest, through a hole in the diaphragm (the muscular sheet separating the chest from the tummy), to the abdomen and then divides into two branches supplying blood to each leg (see left hand panel of of figure 2.1).

Aneurysms or a blow-out in the aorta

The aorta may become enlarged, the wall may weaken and bulge (*aneurysm*) and this may burst (*ruptured aneurysm*). This may occur at its origin in the chest or in the tummy but also in other arteries, for example, the brain arteries. Aneurysms most commonly occur in older people with high blood pressure and also, less commonly, in younger people who have a soft and weak-walled aorta (Marfan's syndrome).

An aneurysm may burst suddenly, causing severe pain in the back if the aneurysm is at the top of the aorta, or in the tummy if the aneurysm is in the abdominal part of the aorta. A burst aneurysm is usually fatal. This is one of the reasons why it is so important that high blood pressure is treated effectively.

Arteries branch off the aorta to supply all parts of the body
(see figure 2.1)

The heart pumps fresh, bright red blood (because it contains a lot of oxygen) through the aorta. Smaller branch arteries (*arterioles*) arise from the aorta and carry fresh blood to the organs and all parts of the body. The arteries divide into smaller and smaller blood vessels. The smallest are called *capillaries*, which are invisible (except with a microscope). Because the walls of capillaries are only one-cell thick, oxygen, nutrients, minerals, and other substances are able to pass out through the thin walls to supply the cells of the body. The used blood containing carbon dioxide and waste products pass back into the capillaries and is then drained back to the heart through another set of blood vessels called *veins*.

How does oxygen move around the body?

Oxygen is attached to a substance in our red blood cells, made of protein and iron, called *hemoglobin*. The oxygen detaches from the hemoglobin when it reaches the cells of the body. If the iron level is low, there is less hemoglobin to carry the oxygen.

Anemia can cause tiredness, breathlessness, and angina – what is it?

Anemia is a low level of hemoglobin. This may be due to blood and iron loss due to heavy periods or bleeding from the gut. The hemoglobin may also be low if there is a low level of vitamins needed for its manufacture. These are folate and vitamin B12. There are other less common causes of anemia related to other diseases.

Very occasionally, severe anemia alone may cause angina because not enough oxygen gets to the heart muscle.

Veins

Veins are soft, thin-walled blood vessels easily seen on the back of the hand, in the arms, in the neck, and in the legs. Blood samples are taken from veins. They carry used, dark purple blood, from all parts of the body back to the right side of the heart. If a vein is cut, the bleeding can be stopped easily by pressing on the cut because the pressure in veins is low (around than 5 mm Hg). Stopping bleeding from a cut artery is much more difficult because the pressure is much higher.

Blood clots and deep vein thromboses (DVTs)

Blood clots can form in veins, most commonly in the veins in the calf (deep vein thrombosis, or DVT). Clots may form if the blood flow in the vein is slow or the blood thickens with dehydration. A DVT causes a hot, painful, and swollen leg. This is treated with painkillers and blood thinners (anticoagulants). Drinking plenty of water to keep the blood thin and liquid, avoiding alcohol (which causes dehydration), not sitting stationary with the legs crossed for long periods, and keeping the legs moving, reduce the risk, particularly on a long air flight. DVTs may also occur in someone who sits or lies in bed for long periods. This is why doctors encourage patients not to stay in bed unless it is really necessary.

Factors Leading to DVTs

- *Obesity*
- *Not moving for a long time (e.g., in bed)*
- *After an operation*
- *Cancer*
- *Thick blood in people who are dehydrated*

Varicose Veins

DVTs are more likely to occur in obese people and if the valves in the veins, which prevent blood falling down to the feet when we stand, have been damaged. This is most common in women

---

who have had several pregnancies. Fault, if incompetent valves can run in families.

DVTs can cause clots in the lungs (pulmonary emboli)

The danger of a DVT is that the blood clot can break free, circulate through the right side of the heart, and then block off the arteries in the lung. In the most extreme case, this can completely stop the circulation, causing death. If no blood can get through the lungs back to the heart, then the circulation stops. It has the same effect as if someone stands on a hosepipe when watering the garden.

In less severe cases, clots in the lungs break up and do not block off the circulation completely. These smaller clots (*pulmonary emboli*) damage the lungs, reducing the amount of oxygen taken up by the lungs. This causes breathlessness and sharp chest pain (*pleurisy*) when the lung and its covering membrane gets damaged and inflamed. Chest infections and pneumonia also inflame the lung lining (pleura), causing pleurisy.

Many of the deaths of people who had heart attacks 50 years ago were not due to a heart problem but to clots in the legs traveling to the lungs (pulmonary emboli). Many of these deaths are now avoided by getting people out of bed and walking around within a day or two of the heart attack.

How is Used Blood Containing Carbon Dioxide Refreshed With Oxygen?

This happens in the lungs. There are two lungs, one on the right and one on the left.

Breathing out stale air containing carbon dioxide. The right side of the heart pumps the stale blood containing carbon dioxide, a by-product of the cells' metabolism, and which is attached to hemoglobin, to the lungs. Here, the carbon dioxide is released through the walls of the very tiny vessels called capillaries. These wrap around the air sacs (alveoli). The carbon dioxide gas travels into the air tubes (*bronchi*) and is then breathed out.

Breathing in oxygen. Around 22% of the air we breathe in is oxygen. Most of the rest is nitrogen. The air containing oxygen travels down the air tubes to the air sacs. The oxygen travels into the capillaries. It then attaches to the hemoglobin in the red cells.

As part of the blood, it travels from the lung blood vessels to the left side of the heart through the pulmonary veins (the only veins in the body carrying fresh oxygen-rich blood).

Gas exchange. The transfer of carbon dioxide out of the capillaries and the entry of oxygen into the blood stream is called gas exchange. It is the main function of the lungs. Smokers get breathless because the chemicals in the tobacco damage the lungs, reducing the amount of lung tissue (*emphysema*) and the ability of the lungs to exchange gas. Any lung condition that reduces the ability of the lung to exchange oxygen for carbon dioxide will cause breathlessness.

The Heart Rate Changes from Minute to Minute Depending on What We Are Doing or Thinking about

In most fit adult people at rest, the heart pumps 70 times in one minute; the heart or pulse rate is therefore 70 beats per minute. It pumps faster during exercise and emotion and slower at rest and when we sleep. The figure of 70 is therefore the average heart rate in most fit adults at rest. Some people have a slower heart rate, because they are fit. It pumps 5 liters of blood per minute around the circulation (that's about 1 small cup of blood every second) and more in a person who is exercising. When necessary, the heart increases its output by beating faster. So, the heart rate may be 50 bpm (beats per minute) when a person is resting but increases to 100 bpm or more when they are active.

Blood pressure changes from minute to minute depending on what we are doing or thinking about. It is important to remember that in the same way as the heart rate speeds up and slows down, from minute to minute, in everyone depending on what they are doing or thinking about, so does the blood pressure. This is why it can be misleading for people to measure their own blood pressure only when they are stressed, tired, worried or have just stopped exercising. GPs and nurses are trained to measure a person's resting blood pressure after the person has been sitting quietly for at least three minutes. It is common and expected for the heart rate to be faster than normal and for the blood pressure to be higher than normal when it is being checked in the GP surgery or in the hospital.

The normal heart rate. The normal heart rate varies between 50–100 bpm. A heart rate slower than this is called *bradycardia*

(slow heart rate) and a heart rate faster than 100 bpm at rest is called *tachycardia.*

A person's maximum heart rate depends on several factors including their age, how fit they are, and what their heart muscle condition is like. A fit young person with a normal heart may have a heart rate at rest of 50 bpm and sometimes less. The heart rate during exercise in a fit, young person may not increase as high as an older unfit person.

How fast can the heart beat? (age predicted maximal heart rate). A person's maximum heart rate during exercise can be estimated by subtracting their age from 220. So the maximum heart rate for an 80-year-old will be $220 - 80 = 140$ bpm; for a 20-year-old, it will be 200 bpm.

Use of a person's age-predicted maximal heart rate. It is useful to know a person's maximal age-predicted heart rate. First, it helps them know if they are exercising close to their maximum (therefore they are doing useful exercise that is good for them and will improve their fitness). Second, we use the maximal heart rate to tell us if a patient has exercised enough or has been sufficiently stressed during an exercise test.

This test is done for several reasons, most commonly in patients with known or suspected coronary heart disease. If we want to see whether a patient may have coronary heart disease and insufficient blood getting to his heart, we exercise him to his age-predicted maximal heart rate. If he does not get angina or develop changes in the electrical recording of the heart (ECG), this suggests that there is enough blood and oxygen getting to their heart and, therefore, the heart arteries are probably not narrowed.

Some people become unnecessarily concerned about their heart rate. Most heart rate monitors in the gym are not very accurate. The most accurate way to count your heart rate is by feeling it at the wrist or with an ECG during a stress test.

How is the heart rate controlled? The heart rate and the blood pressure are constantly changing from minute to minute depending on what we are doing or thinking about. The normal heart rate (pulse rate) ranges between 50–100 bpm. The average heart would contract 3 million times per year! That is a lot of squeezing during a life of 80 years or more. Unlike our arm and leg muscles, which are made from a different type of muscle,

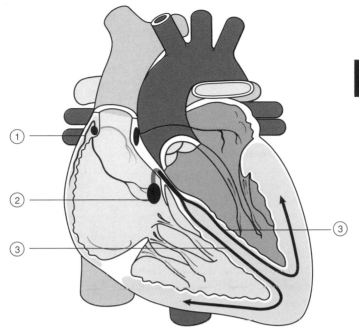

2

Figure 2.4: The electrical conducting system (electrical wiring) of the heart. (1): Electrical impulses from the pacemaker in the right collecting chamber (right atrium) travel to (2) a junction box (the atrioventricular node) above the two ventricles (pumping chambers). (3) The electrical impulses then travel in the muscles of the right and left ventricles in special "bundles" of cells.

our heart cannot take a complete rest when the rest of our body sleeps. Otherwise, we would not wake up!

The heart's inbuilt pacemaker sets the heart rate and is controlled by other nerves. The heart rate is controlled by special cells called the *pacemaker* (the sinus node). It is situated in the right collecting chamber. It is called the pacemaker because it sends out electrical impulses at a rate faster than other parts of the heart muscle, all of which also send out impulses. The pacemaker impulses are quicker and so suppress or inhibit the impulses coming from other parts of the heart.

These electrical signals stimulate or trigger the heart muscle to contract, and pump.

1 Electrical impulses from the heart's pacemaker (special cells in the wall of the right collecting chamber – the right atrium),

travel to the "junction box" – the atrioventricular node (2), which is between the two collecting chambers and the two pumping chambers.

2. The electrical impulses then travel in the muscle of the two pumping chambers (the left and right ventricles) causing the muscle cells to contract. This results in the heart contracting (squeezing) and pumping blood around the body (circulation of blood).

Missed or extra beats. Many people complain of palpitation as if their heart "misses a beat" or they may feel an extra beat. Some people feel that on occasions, their heart is racing or beating forcefully. Most commonly, this is due to anxiety and stress and this also occurs, normally, with exertion. The most reliable way to find out if the fast heart rate is normal or due to an abnormal heart rhythm is to record an ECG during an attack.

Palpitation is an awareness of your heartbeat. The most common palpitations are due to extra beats coming from the collecting or pumping chamber in their heart. They are usually harmless. They come from parts of the heart outside the usual conducting system (ectopic = out of place, as in ectopic pregnancy). They reset the heart's pacemaker.

An extra or ectopic beat occurs earlier than the normal beat and may not be felt. After the ectopic beat, there is a slight delay during which the heart has longer to fill. When the next normal beat occurs, after the slight pause, there is more blood to be squeezed out and this may be felt as an "extra beat."

The Sympathetic and Parasympathetic Nervous Systems

The *sympathetic nervous system* speeds the heart up and also increases the blood pressure. It makes us feel excited and our hands sweaty, due to release of adrenaline and noradrenaline.

The *parasympathetic nervous system* slows the heart down. The parasympathetic system comes into play when we are resting, after we've eaten a big meal, and when we are sleeping.

Problems with the heart rate

A *slow heart rate* can cause breathlessness, heart failure, dizzy spells, or loss of consciousness.

A *fast heart rate* can cause an unpleasant awareness of the heart beat (palpitation), chest pain, breathlessness, dizzy spells, and loss of consciousness.

When are artificial pacemakers put in?

When the heart rate is very slow (less than 40 beats per minute) and if people lose consciousness or feel dizzy due to a slow heart rate, a pacemaker is put in. Pacemakers are now also being put in to improve the function of a weak heart in patients with severe heart failure. There are also special pacemakers called implantable cardiac defibrillators, which are put in patients who have dangerous heart rhythms.

Angina

Read this chapter to learn about:

- angina, what it is, what it feels like and what causes it
- the other causes of chest pain that can feel like angina
- what to do if you get angina
- what tests are done for patients with angina
- what treatments are given to patients with angina

ANGINA: WHAT DOES IT FEEL LIKE?

- Angina is an uncomfortable feeling in the chest, occurring during exercise or stress, when the heart beats faster and works harder. Angina is due to a lack of blood and oxygen getting to the heart muscle caused by blocked heart arteries.
- It is commonly described as a tightness, a squeezing sensation, a burning feeling or a pressure or heaviness in the chest. Most patients do not complain of pain.
- It can spread to the shoulders, neck, jaw, arms, or upper tummy. Some people feel it only in one or more of these areas. It may spread to the arm, the throat, or the jaw. People who get angina only in the jaw think that they have "toothache" and may go to see their dentist.
- It lasts only a few minutes. It fades away when the patient rests or if the stress goes away. It usually goes away quickly after a puff or two of an anti-anginal spray (glyceryl trinitrate spray).

What Types of Pain Make Angina Unlikely?

The following types of sensation are not angina:

- a pricking, sharp, knife-like, pulsating, dagger-through-the-chest feeling
- a pain that comes on or goes away in certain body positions

- symptoms that come on at random times and not related to exercise

> *A pricking feeling in the chest or a stabbing pain in the nipple or under the left breast is very rarely, if ever, due to angina.*

Does Angina Make Your Chest Sore or Tender to the Touch?

No. Angina never causes tenderness of the chest wall. If the chest wall or ribs are tender, and pressing over the tender spot duplicates the pain, then it is not angina. A chest wall problem or a rib problem is much more likely.

Is Pain "over the Heart Area" Likely to Be Angina?

It depends on what the pain is like and when it occurs. Even though the heart lies just to the left of the breastbone (sternum), angina is not felt within a small area; it is not localized to one spot. Angina can be felt anywhere in the chest.

Can Angina Last for Hours?

Rarely. Angina usually lasts for less than 20 minutes. If it lasts more than 20 minutes, the discomfort is severe, the person is sweaty, very breathless, and feels faint, sick and awful, he may be having a heart attack. He should call an ambulance and go to hospital immediately.

DO WOMEN GET ANGINA IN THE SAME WAY AS MEN?

Not always. Angina in women is more unusual and this makes it more difficult to diagnose angina in women.

For example, women have more variation in the amount of exercise they can do before getting angina. They may get attacks of angina at night and at rest more commonly than men.

Women get attacks of chest pain more commonly than men, but most of these attacks are not due to angina. They often complain of a pricking sensation under the left breast. If this is not related to exertion or stress, it is unlikely to be due to angina.

Women are more likely than men to have angina but normal heart arteries.

WHY DOES ANGINA OCCUR?

Angina occurs when there is not enough blood and oxygen getting to the heart muscle. This is because the heart (coronary) arteries are narrowed or blocked (figure 1.2).

In the same way as a car engine needs more fuel when we want to accelerate, so the heart needs more blood when it beats faster and more forcefully when we exercise or get stressed.

SITUATIONS THAT MAY CAUSE ANGINA

- **Walking fast, rushing and exercising**
  Some patients notice angina when walking fast or uphill. Many people notice angina more when walking after a meal. This is because after eating, blood is diverted away from the heart to the stomach for digestion. This decreases the amount of blood available for the heart to do its work. This can be confusing for patients and doctors because patients may think they are suffering from indigestion and not a heart problem. Indigestion may feel very similar to angina. Angina is also more common in winter because the heart has to work harder to pump blood around the arteries, which narrow down in the cold weather.
- **Stress and emotion**
  Angina is also felt by some people when they are stressed or anxious, commonly when watching sports or a frightening film, because the heart rate and the blood pressure increase.

Typical angina:

- *chest discomfort, pressure, or heaviness sometimes spreading to the arms or throat*
- *shortness of breath*
- *occurring with exercise or stress*
- *lasting a few minutes and fading away*

WHAT SORT OF PEOPLE GET ANGINA?

Angina is more likely to occur in:

- the elderly
- smokers
- people with a high cholesterol level, particularly the "bad" LDL (low density lipoprotein) cholesterol
- people with high blood pressure
- diabetics
- people with a low blood count (anemia)
- people with an overactive thyroid gland
- people who are overweight or obese and have a high fat diet
- people who do not exercise regularly
- people who are stressed or depressed.

If a person has at least one of the characteristics listed above and has chest symptoms that could fit with angina, he probably has angina and, therefore, coronary heart disease.

Can Young People Get Angina?

Yes, but it is unusual in people under 40 years of age unless they have risk factors for coronary heart disease.

Nowadays, most people with angina are over 60, although some young people may get it. It affects men and women equally although it affects women when they are older. Angina symptoms have different characteristics in women (atypical angina). We do not understand why. It may have something to do with female hormones. This is controversial because hormone replacement treatment (HRT) does not protect women from coronary heart disease and angina.

Does Everyone with Narrowed or Blocked Heart Arteries Get Angina?

No. Some people with blocked arteries do not get angina. The first sign may be a heart attack or sudden death. It is not understood why some people do not get warnings. Some might, but dismiss it as indigestion. Symptoms depend on a person's lifestyle. For example, an elderly person may have narrowed heart

---

arteries, but because they don't exercise or move around, they do not get angina.

Diabetics may have narrowed heart arteries, but may not get angina. It is thought that their diabetes affects the way nerve impulses from the heart are recognized by the brain.

Some People with Bad Heart Arteries May Get Breathless Rather Than Get Chest Discomfort

Breathlessness may be angina and not due to lung disease or being unfit. People with a lack of oxygen to the heart may feel short of breath when rushing around or during exercise because if the heart does not get enough oxygen, there is a build-up of fluid in the lungs. Therefore, if you are more breathless than you think you should be, see your doctor. Apart from being unfit and overweight or having lung disease, a chest infection, or asthma, your breathlessness may be angina.

IS IT TRUE THAT THE WORSE THE ANGINA, THE WORSE THE HEART ARTERIES?

Yes, most of the time. But many people with bad angina have surprisingly good arteries and many people with very bad arteries have no angina at all. For example, 50% of people with coronary heart disease have no angina, and the first they "know" about it is when they have a heart attack or die from a heart attack. The other 50% of people with coronary heart disease may get very severe angina, whereas others whose coronary arteries are just as bad may get only very mild, occasional attacks, and only when doing very vigorous exercise.

Therefore, there is an inconsistent relationship between symptoms and the severity of coronary heart disease.

For reasons that are not understood, some people appear to have a "defective anginal warning system" or a "numb heart." The elderly and diabetics are well known to have this condition. During a routine examination or before they have a non-cardiac operation (for example, a hip replacement), the electrical recording of the heart (ECG) may show the signs of a past heart attack. They are often surprised when asked about this and reply "what heart attack? I haven't had a heart attack!" Heart attacks may be silent. This is because a large proportion of patients do not feel angina and do not feel the symptoms of a heart attack.

Is It More Dangerous to Have All Three Arteries Narrowed or Blocked Than Only One?

Yes. And it also matters where the artery is blocked. It is more dangerous if the artery is blocked at the origin or top end of the artery, because less blood gets to the heart.

Some People Die Suddenly from a Heart Attack without Having Had Angina: Why?

A heart attack occurs if one of the three heart arteries blocks off (*coronary thrombosis*).

For many people with coronary heart disease, their first symptom is a heart attack or sudden death, without ever having had any warning symptoms of angina.

Heart attacks are very dangerous and unpredictable. 30% of patients die before reaching hospital. The sudden lack of blood and oxygen to the heart causes a fatal heart rhythm called *ventricular fibrillation*; the heart stops beating and the circulation of blood around the body stops. Even with prompt medical care and attempts to resuscitate the patient, these attacks are usually fatal.

The other half of patients recover from their heart attack. Modern medical treatments continue to improve the chances of a longer, more active life for survivors of heart attacks.

IS ANGINA A "KILLER"?

It depends on the age of the patient, what his heart arteries are like and how badly they are narrowed, how strong his heart is and whether he has other serious medical conditions.

> *Many people live with stable angina for many years and do not die from a heart attack, but from a completely different condition at a ripe old age. However, it should be remembered that the risk of death from heart attacks or stroke increases as we get older.*

Angina can be stable for many years, producing little or no problems, but for unknown reasons becomes unstable and causes a heart attack.

WHAT IS STABLE ANGINA?

Angina that occurs while doing a certain amount of exercise under certain conditions is called *stable angina*. It occurs predictably and consistently. For example, people know that if they walk up a steep hill quickly, into a cold wind, or soon after a heavy meal, or if they do too much housework or get too excited, they will get chest discomfort. Patients with stable angina can predict that their symptoms will occur when they do certain things and can stop before this happens. Stable angina would be expected to occur if their heart has to work above a certain level. It is similar to a car running smoothly and accelerating up to 70 mph but if pushed to 90 mph, the car vibrates and the engine does not sound right because it is trying to generate more power than it can comfortably produce.

What Should You Do if You Get Angina while Doing Normal Things?

Stop what you are doing, rest, and take a glyceryl trinitrate (GTN) spray or tablet if you wish. The angina should disappear quickly. If you notice that your angina is getting more frequent and occurring at a lower level of activity, see your doctor. Your stable angina may be developing into unstable angina. You may need more medication or some heart tests.

Is It Dangerous to Take More Than One Puff of GTN Spray?

No. You can take two puffs. Some people get a headache with GTN and don't like taking it. Some people feel light-headed. Very occasionally, some people black out after taking a lot of GTN because it lowers blood pressure.

WHAT IS UNSTABLE ANGINA?

It can take different forms:

- angina occurring for the first time (new angina)
- an increase in the number of attacks (worsening of angina in someone who has had angina for some time),
- angina attacks occurring when doing very little exercise or, worse still, when at rest.

For example, a patient may have been able to mow the lawn or make the beds without getting angina. If doing these things, she begins to notice chest pain, then her angina has become unstable. She can no longer do what she did before.

Unstable angina is more dangerous than stable angina. It means that the person is at increased risk of having a heart attack. Patients may get very worried and anxious when their angina does not go away when they use their GTN spray. This can be alarming and patients should see their doctor, or if their angina lasts for more than 20 minutes and is more severe than usual, they should go directly to the hospital in case they are having a heart attack.

IF I HAVE UNSTABLE ANGINA, WHAT SHOULD I DO?

Contact your doctor or go straight to the hospital for assessment and treatment. You may be advised to stay in the hospital to make sure that you are not in the early stages of a heart attack.

Why Does Stable Angina Become Unstable?

This is not known. Something makes the inner lining of the artery inflamed.

Are the Arteries Different in Patients with Stable and Unstable Angina?

Yes. The arteries in patients with *unstable angina* are usually more narrowed but are also inflamed. There may be small blood clots in the artery, which can block off completely. The blood clots form where an unstable lump of soft fat (unstable plaque) has cracked open. The patient feels angina due to the blocked artery preventing blood flow to the heart.

The heart arteries in patients with *stable angina* are narrowed with a hard type of fat (atheroma) but are not inflamed and the top surface of the fatty lump (*plaque*) is firm and hard and less likely to crack open (stable plaque).

Is It Possible to Have Angina with Normal Heart Arteries?

Yes, but this is rare. Nearly all people who have angina have coronary heart disease.

What Medical Conditions Cause Angina in People with Normal Heart Arteries?

People can get angina even though they have normal heart arteries and have a normal blood supply to their heart muscle. These conditions are:

- A narrowed aortic outflow valve in the left side of the heart, which can cause thickening of the heart muscle. Many people with a narrowed outflow valve also have blocked arteries because the risk factors are the same for each condition (the things that increase the chances of getting coronary heart disease also increase the chances of having a narrowed aortic valve).
- Severe thickening of the walls of the heart. This is most commonly due to high blood pressure (hypertension). Less commonly, it may be due to a condition called *hypertrophic cardiomyopathy*, which is sometimes passed on in families, and where the blood pressure is normal. In these conditions where the heart muscle is thick, it is not the *supply* of blood and oxygen to the heart muscle that is abnormal, but its *distribution in the heart muscle cells*, which are big and distorted.
- Very high pressure in the lung arteries (pulmonary arterial hypertension, a very rare condition).

ANGINA AND NORMAL CORONARY ARTERIES: "SYNDROME X"

Less commonly, some people may have angina but are found to have normal heart arteries. We do not understand the reasons for this. They also have an abnormal ECG during exercise (exercise stress test). This combination is called "syndrome X." The cause is not known (that's why it's called syndrome X), but unlike angina due to narrowed arteries, it generally causes no problems in the future and is treated with tablets. Although patients may get chest pain occasionally, it cannot be treated with angioplasty or heart bypass surgery, because the arteries are normal. Patients can be reassured that they are, despite the episodes of chest pain, at low risk of dying from a heart attack.

WHAT ARE THE OTHER CAUSES OF CHEST PAIN?

There are several causes of chest pain other than angina. Apart from the heart, there are other important parts of the body situated in the chest that may cause chest pain. These are the gut, the lungs, and the chest wall and spine.

Chest Pain May Also Be Due to Problems with:

- the gullet (esophagus – the food tube in the throat)
- the stomach
- the duodenum (the part of the gut after the stomach)
- the gallbladder
- the lungs, and the membrane lining around the lungs (pleura)
- the chest wall – skin, ribs, muscle, cartilages joining the ribs to the breastbone (sternum)
- the large artery coming out of the heart called the aorta. All the other arteries branch off this most important artery
- the neck (cervical spine).

Common Causes of Chest Pain Not Due to Angina

- Indigestion

This is a burning pain felt in the middle of the chest behind the breastbone. It may occur after eating or during a meal. Some people feel a bitter, acid taste in their mouth due to acid from the stomach spilling back (refluxing) up the gullet. Some people belch a lot. This can be because they eat too much, too quickly. Hot, spicy food may also cause indigestion and chest pain. Chest pain occurring in bed at night is often due to reflux of acid and other contents from the stomach.

It is often very difficult to know whether a person has angina or indigestion and tests are often necessary to distinguish the two conditions. Both conditions may respond to a GTN spray. It is important to make sure that the person does not have coronary heart disease. It is also not uncommon for people to have both indigestion and angina, and both conditions will need treating.

A *hiatus hernia* is a common cause of indigestion. It is due to part of the stomach being pushed up from the tummy

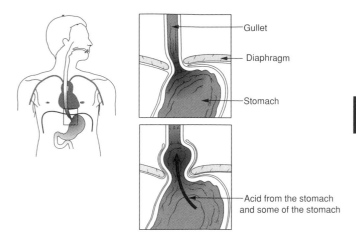

Figure 3.1: Hiatus hernia: Acid can reflux back up from the stomach, up the gullet (oesophagus), causing heartburn, belching, and indigestion. A hiatus is a gap or hole in the muscular sheet called the diaphragm, which separates the chest from the tummy (abdomen). If the hiatus is big enough, some of the stomach acid refluxes up the gullet, causing inflammation of the lining of the gullet. This causes pain, acidity, and gas and can be confused with a heart attack or angina.

through the hole in the partition sheet (the diaphragm) into the chest. The stomach acid burns the inside of the gullet.

Indigestion is common in pregnancy and in overweight people, because the stomach is squeezed and acid from the stomach is pushed back into the gullet.

Indigestion improves after delivery of the baby. It also improves when overweight people lose weight, eat smaller meals, and do not go to bed on a full stomach.

The condition is treated with medicine to neutralize the acid (antacids), and tablets to decrease the amount of acid secreted by the stomach. Chest pain may also be caused by ulcers in the stomach and duodenum. These can be treated with tablets.

Occasionally, an inflamed and infected gallbladder causes not only severe tummy pain, nausea, vomiting, and fever (*cholecystitis* – an inflamed and infected gallbladder), but severe chest pain. In severe cases, the gallbladder needs to be removed.

How Are Indigestion and Heartburn Diagnosed?

The diagnosis is made from what the patient tells the doctor.

Sometimes it is helpful to look at the inside of the gullet and stomach using a fiberoptic tube (endoscope) put down the gullet through the mouth. Samples of the stomach juices are taken because the condition may be due to an infection (*Helicobacter pylori*) that can be cured with antibiotics and other tablets. In the elderly and in people who have lost weight or lost their appetite, cancer has to be considered.

Lung Causes of Chest Pain

- **Pain from the lungs**
  Pleurisy is a sharp pain in the chest made worse when the patient breathes deeply. It is due to inflammation of the lining around the lungs (the pleura). This is most commonly caused by a chest infection (pneumonia) and less commonly, by a clot in the lungs (pulmonary embolus).
- **Pain arising from the chest wall**
  The chest wall is made of skin, muscle, bone, and cartilages and there are nerves and blood vessels running in the grooves at the bottom of the ribs. Chest pain may come from any of these parts of the chest wall.

  Muscular pain is unpleasant and can be caused as a result of a fall, a sports injury, lifting something heavy, or an accident. It usually gets better on its own but can take a long time.

  Rib pain due to a broken rib may occur after a fall, a car accident, or a sports injury. It is very painful and restricts all kinds of movements. It can, for example, be very difficult to get out of bed or a chair. Sometimes, elderly women with thin or brittle bones (*osteoporosis*) may get rib fractures for no apparent reason. Sometimes, the fractured rib may tear the membrane lining around the lungs causing collapse of the lung (*pneumothorax*). Depending on how much lung has collapsed, it can cause breathlessness and can be painful. A tube may have to be inserted into the lung to suck out the air and allow the lung to expand.

  Shingles can be a painful skin condition caused by the chickenpox virus. It causes severe, continuous pain and a rash. Occasionally, the pain from the skin may last a long time despite treatment.

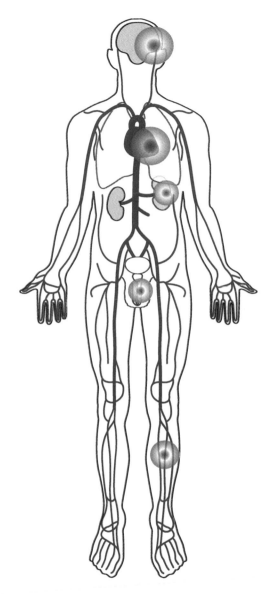

- **The aorta**

  The aorta is the largest artery in the body. It extends from the heart, up to the upper chest, and then turns sharply down through the diaphragm to the lower tummy, where it divides into two branches to supply each leg.

Arteries branch off it to all parts of the body. A tear in the aorta (dissection of the aorta) is very serious and often fatal. Blood pours out of the aorta and the victim bleeds to death quickly. Sometimes, there is a slow tear from the top or bottom of the aorta and these can be repaired. Tears in the aorta occur most commonly in elderly men who have high blood pressure (and other cardiovascular risk factors). This is one of the reasons why it is so important for everyone to have normal blood pressure.

The site of pain due to a tear (dissection) of the aorta depends on where the tear is. A tear in the top part of the aorta in the chest feels as if you have been stabbed in the back. A torn aorta in the tummy (ruptured abdominal aorta) causes severe pain in the tummy, collapse, and loss of consciousness. If the tear does not seal itself, it is fatal within a few minutes, unless emergency surgery is possible.

- The neck
  Pain in the chest may come from a trapped nerve in the neck due to arthritis in the spine. The pain can be severe and patients may also have pins and needles, numbness, and funny feelings in their fingers and arms. This is because the nerves supplying the arms and hands come out from between the bones in the neck.

- Anxiety
  Sometimes no cause can be found for a person's chest pain, despite doing tests for all the conditions listed above. Many people are born worriers and worry that they may have a heart problem. Others may have a friend or a family member who has a serious heart problem, and they are anxious that they may have a similar condition.

  Tests may need to be done to be able to reassure them and their family that their heart is in good condition and strong, and that they have nothing serious to worry about. Often, reassurance is effective and their symptoms and anxiety are relieved.

WHAT SHOULD I DO IF I THINK I AM GETTING ANGINA?

First, see your doctor to make sure that it is angina rather than something else. The doctor may want to do some tests or refer you to a specialist or alternatively, start you on treatment and monitor your progress.

How Does a Doctor Know if Someone Has Angina?

A doctor knows only from the person's description of his symptoms. We call this a clinical diagnosis.

Although we can do tests to see if a patient has coronary heart disease, angina is diagnosed from what the patient tells us, and not by a test. That is why it is so important for the patient to describe to the doctor what he feels and for the doctor to listen very carefully to the patient's symptoms.

DOES EVERYONE WITH CORONARY HEART DISEASE GET ANGINA?

No. Perhaps only half the patients who have coronary heart disease get angina. The reason for this is not understood. This is why a lot of people who have had a heart attack, and so have coronary heart disease, had no warnings of angina. Sometimes, a person's angina disappears after he has had a heart attack.

So just because a patient has coronary heart disease does not mean that he has angina. Having coronary heart disease does not mean that a person needs angioplasty or heart bypass. He may need tablets.

IS IT DANGEROUS TO BE ACTIVE, DO EXERCISE OR HAVE SEX IF YOU HAVE ANGINA?

Not unless you have unstable angina. Some people may first notice angina during exercise or sex. If you do, see your doctor.

Exercising in the cold, walking into a cold winter wind, or doing winter sports, particularly at high altitude, can be dangerous to people with bad angina. Elderly people who live in cold homes may notice that their angina is worse in winter.

For most people with stable angina, exercise is not only safe but beneficial. It is generally best to avoid rushing around, and you should try to avoid stressful situations. However, modern treatment of angina is not about wrapping patients up in cotton wool, preventing them from living a full and active life

Nowadays, we encourage people with angina to get out and about, to play sports, have an active social and sexual life, and do everything they would want to do. It is important to make sure that:

- Angina rather than another condition is the cause of the chest symptom.
- Patients do everything possible to reduce the chances of the arteries getting blocked and therefore reduce their risk of having a heart attack. This will usually involve major changes to their lifestyle.
- Patients understand that they may need to take tablets long term.
- An invasive X-ray test of the heart arteries (coronary angiogram) and other procedures or operations may be necessary depending on how severe the symptoms are and what the heart arteries are like. The patient's views on what he wants are very important.
- Patients take a GTN spray or pill before doing anything that might cause angina.

Exercise has been shown to be more effective than angioplasty in patients with stable angina and single vessel coronary artery disease.

Can I Continue to Work if I Have Angina?

Yes, unless you are an airline pilot. Some car and taxi drivers may be barred if they have an abnormal exercise test result. People who do a stressful job may need to modify their work and avoid doing the things that make cause angina. This may be very difficult.

What about Driving?

You can drive as long as your angina is stable, but you should inform your car insurance company. You may need a letter from your doctor stating that it is safe for you to continue driving. You should stop driving if you get angina while driving.

There are also rules for people who drive public service vehicles, like buses, subways, and trains.

Is Flying Safe if You Have Angina?

Yes, unless the patient has unstable angina. The amount of oxygen in the cabin may fall and is a little lower when the plane is at its flight altitude. The lower oxygen level can upset some people and trigger angina. People with unstable angina should not fly, but it is generally safe for people with stable angina to fly.

Remember to take enough pills, plan your vacation, and if you cannot carry your suitcase, try to get some help. If you are worried about getting on board the plane, train, or ship, you may be able to get a wheelchair with the help of a doctor's letter.

KEEPING AN EYE ON PATIENTS WITH CORONARY HEART DISEASE

Coronary heart disease is not curable, even with heart bypass (the patient doesn't change; the arteries are bypassed and the arteries or veins used as bypasses can get blocked up). So we need to monitor the patient over the long term to decide whether we need to change treatment, to monitor and control risk factors, and encourage the patient to lead a full and active life. New treatments for heart disease come along all the time. It is helpful for patients to see their doctor so that they may get the benefit of new treatments and advice.

SO HOW DO DOCTORS FIND OUT IF PEOPLE HAVE CORONARY HEART DISEASE?

GPs are encouraging their patients to visit them for checks on blood pressure, weight, cholesterol, and blood sugar. Doctors and nurses help patients stop smoking and give advice about diet, exercise, and lifestyle. These checks help identify patients at risk. Patients with chest pain, who may have ignored their symptoms, have the opportunity to tell the doctor about their symptoms.

Very often, impotence may be the first sign of arterial disease. Men who are impotent should discuss this with their doctor, even if it is not a problem.

Chest discomfort and breathlessness occurring during exercise or stress in a patient who has one or more cardiovascular risk factors is probably angina. These patients may need further tests, treatment, or referral to a specialist.

Is it possible to know whether or not someone has coronary heart disease without doing any special tests?

Yes.

There are two examples of someone at low risk and someone at high risk.

1. A young, fit person, less than 50 years old, who has no angina and no cardiovascular risk factors, would, 99 times out of 100, have normal heart arteries.

2. A person, who has definitely had a heart attack, would have coronary heart disease with at least some blockage in one of the three heart arteries. The artery may not necessarily be blocked because some people, particularly young people, may have a heart attack and the blocked heart artery may open up by itself soon afterwards.

3. Virtually everyone (98%) with angina has some coronary heart disease.

What Tests Are Done for Patients with Angina?

Even if a person has definite angina, it may not be necessary to do any tests, at least immediately, unless the angina is severe. People with unstable angina should be referred promptly for a specialist's opinion.

- Blood pressure and blood tests
  It is important to see your GP who may check your blood pressure, check your pulse, do some blood tests (sugar, cholesterol, blood count, and kidney function), and an ECG.

- Electrocardiogram
  This will identify patients who have had a heart attack in the past. If the ECG is recorded while the patient is having chest pain, the ECG may show abnormalities that confirm the diagnosis that the symptoms are due to the heart and not indigestion (figure 3.2).

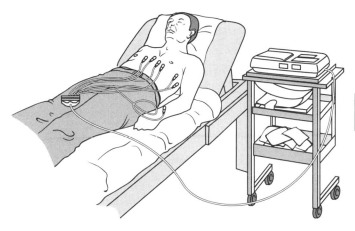

Figure 3.2: ECG: Diagram of an ECG (electrocardiogram), a tracing of the electrical activity of the heart.

Tests Should Be Done Only If the Results Help the Doctor Decide What the Best Treatment Is for That Patient.

If a patient has definite angina that is interfering with his life, then the GP may start the patient on pills. Depending on the patient, the GP may refer the patient to a cardiologist for tests.

What Test Is Done if It Is Not Clear That the Patient Has Angina?

Exercise testing is usually done as a first step to confirm that the patient has a lack of blood supply to his heart. It may be necessary to do a coronary angiogram to show what the heart arteries look like, or the patient may initially be given pills.

Accuracy of Heart Tests: Does an Abnormal Test Result Always Mean That Something Is Wrong or Abnormal?

No. Although some tests tell us whether a person has a condition or not, for example, a pregnancy test, a blood count, or a blood sugar test, other tests are not perfect and have to be interpreted with caution.

Exercise tests and stress echocardiography tell us the *proba bility* that a patient has coronary heart disease. The only accurate

---

Angina   **61**

way to tell if a patient definitely has coronary heart disease, or blockages in a heart artery is with a coronary angiogram.

WHY IS EXERCISE USED TO STRESS THE HEART IN A PATIENT WITH ANGINA?

Exercise tests are done to see if a patient has enough oxygen getting to his heart. It tells us how likely it is (the probability) that a patient has coronary heart disease. Exercise is used to provoke a problem, to try to reproduce what patients feel when they exercise or exert themselves and increase their heart rate.

Exercise is a way to stress the heart by getting the patient to cycle or walk fast on a treadmill. The faster the heart beats and the higher the pressure it generates in order to push blood around the body to the muscles of the legs (the biggest muscles in the body), the more oxygen it needs. If the heart has a normal blood supply (the heart arteries are normal), then the patient should not get any angina while exercising and there should be no changes in the electrical recording of the heart (ECG) during the test (true negative).

A patient with blocked heart arteries may get chest discomfort and there may also be abnormalities in the ECG (true positive).

IS IT SAFE TO EXERCISE A PATIENT WHO MAY HAVE A HEART PROBLEM?

Yes, unless the patient is having a heart attack or has unstable angina. But the doctor would make sure that the patient did not have these before requesting the test.

DOES AN EXERCISE TEST TELL US WHETHER OR NOT A PATIENT HAS CORONARY HEART DISEASE?

Most of the time, yes, but the result has to be interpreted carefully, with knowledge of the patient's condition.

When comparing the result to that of a coronary angiogram, there are four different possible results from an exercise test.

- Most people (80%) who have coronary heart disease will have an abnormality on their exercise test (true positive).

- Most people (80%) who have normal heart arteries will have a normal exercise test result (true negative).
- Some people (20%) with coronary heart disease may have a normal exercise test result (false negative).
- Some people (20%) who have completely normal heart arteries may have an abnormal exercise test result (false positive).

FALSE POSITIVE TESTS: THE PERSON IS NORMAL BUT THE TEST IS ABNORMAL

Around 20% of people who have normal heart arteries may have an abnormal test result with an abnormal ECG. Often, an experienced cardiologist will be able to tell if the type of ECG abnormality is likely to be a false positive by examining the whole recording and seeing the patient.

False positive ECG recordings during exercise are quite common in young people, particularly females, and can be due to them breathing heavily and fast (hyperventilation), and also in people with a thickened heart muscle, due to high blood pressure.

False positive results can cause anxiety in both the patient and the doctor. An abnormal test result in a person, who is unlikely to have coronary heart disease, should be viewed with suspicion.

FALSE NEGATIVE TESTS: THE PATIENT IS ABNORMAL BUT THE TEST IS NORMAL

A false negative exercise test means that the patient would be expected to have an abnormal test result because he has coronary heart disease, but the test result is negative (normal).

A Man with Coronary Heart Disease but a Normal Exercise Test Result

An example of a "false negative" test result would be of a 65-year-old man who has typical angina and an almost "full house" of cardiovascular risk factors (he smokes, he is very overweight, he has a high cholesterol level, and he has high blood pressure and diabetes). When he does the exercise test, there are no ECG changes and he does not get angina. This test is almost certainly wrong and misleading. The fact that he has angina means that he has at least a 95% chance of having coronary heart disease, even ignoring his risk factors.

EXERCISE TESTING

This is done on a bicycle (like the ones in the gym) or a treadmill. Patients have to be able and willing to do the test. The purpose of an exercise test is to stress the heart by getting the patient to increase his heart rate and blood pressure. The aim is to see whether during exercise, there is enough blood getting to the heart muscle. If there isn't, this suggests that the heart arteries are blocked or narrowed. The test is also useful because it measures how much exercise the patient can do, what happens to his heart rate and blood pressure during exercise, and whether he gets chest discomfort or breathlessness during the test.

Exercise testing is also very helpful in patients who have had a heart attack and if done before they leave hospital, saves the patient the anxiety of doing his own unsupervised exercise test at home. The result can be used to advise patients how much they can and should exercise (exercise prescription).

Most patients who have at least one of their three main heart arteries blocked or narrowed will develop an abnormality.

THINGS WE LOOK FOR FROM AN EXERCISE TEST:

- Does the patient experience chest pain or undue breathlessness during exercise?
- How much exercise (measured in minutes) can the patient do? The more, the better, and the better his prognosis (how he fares in the future).
- Does the patient develop any changes in the ECG during exercise?
- What are the patient's heart rate and blood pressure at their peak?
- How quickly does the patient recover? The heart rate should fall by at least 20 beats per minute within one minute of stopping.
- Are there any heart rhythm abnormalities? These indicate that problems may occur over the next few years.

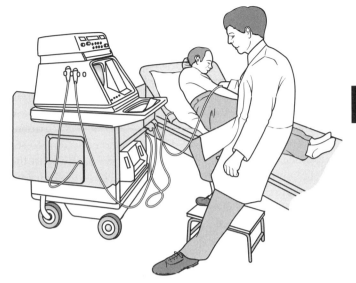

Figure 3.3: Diagram of heart ultrasound (echocardiogram) being performed.

Exercise Stress Ultrasound (Echocardiography)

This is sometimes used if the patient has an ECG that is difficult to interpret, for example, a problem in the conduction of electricity in the heart's conduction system (bundle branch block). Patients do an exercise test and have an ECG to measure their heart rate, but at the end of the exercise test, an ultrasound test of their heart is done to see if any parts of the heart are not working normally. Parts of the heart muscle that do not get enough blood during exercise do not work (squeeze down or contract) properly. These parts of the heart can be seen on the ultrasound (figure 3.3).

Exercise Stress Ultrasound Is Not Perfect Because:

- There are 15% false positives and 15% false negative test results.
- It is not possible to get good-quality pictures of the heart in all patients.

Dobutamine Stress Ultrasound (Echocardiography)

Dobutamine is a drug given to patients who have a very weak heart and heart failure. It increases the power of the heart. It has to be injected slowly (infused) and cannot be given as a pill. It works by increasing the heart rate and blood pressure and so has similar effects as exercise. It is used in patients who cannot exercise, for example, those with weak legs or who are too old to exercise.

Patients lie on a couch and dobutamine is infused through a "drip" tube in a vein in the back of their hand or arm. The dose of dobutamine is gradually increased to increase the heart rate and blood pressure.

It is interpreted in the same way as if the patient had an exercise stress echocardiogram.

Dobutamine Stress Ultrasound Is Not Perfect Because:

- There are 15% false positives and 15% false negative test results.

SHOULD EVERYONE WHO HAS CHEST PAIN HAVE A STRESS TEST?

No. These tests are most helpful in people who are at intermediate risk of having coronary heart disease. They are less useful of people who are either very likely, or very unlikely, to have coronary heart disease.

- **People at high risk of having coronary heart disease**
  Virtually all patients with angina and those who have had a heart attack have coronary heart disease. This is because they would not have angina, and would not have had a heart attack, unless they had narrowed heart arteries. Only very occasionally do we see patients, most commonly middle-aged females, who have angina but normal coronary arteries.

  It is likely that these patients will have an abnormal exercise test result. If they do, it is not a surprise. If they have a normal test result, it will probably be a false negative.

  In these patients, we do not do heart tests to find out if they have coronary heart disease because we already know that they do. Tests may be done to see how severe the condition is. This helps us decide on the best treatment.

- **People at low risk of having coronary heart disease**

  These are typically young people with no angina and who have no risk factors. They may have chest symptoms for reasons other than a heart problem. Sometimes, particularly in anxious patients, cardiac tests are done to exclude heart problems and to reassure them. An abnormal ECG recording is most likely to be a false positive response and therefore can be confusing.

- **Intermediate risk of coronary heart disease**

  Exercise tests are most helpful in this group of patients. They are neither at low risk or at high risk, but in between.

  They may have chest symptoms that are difficult to pin down as angina, or one or more cardiovascular risk factors.

What you should do whether or not you have coronary heart disease

- Stop smoking completely. Even one cigarette a day increases the risk of a heart attack.
- Make sure your cholesterol is low.
- Get slim and stay slim.
- Have a low fat, low salt, low carbohydrate diet.
- Exercise for 30 minutes every day.
- Identify the cause of your stress and do something effective about it.
- Make sure your blood pressure is normal.
- Make sure your blood sugar is normal and that you do not have diabetes.

DIET AND ANGINA

People who are overweight should try their hardest to achieve their ideal weight and shape. They should have a healthy, very low fat and low carbohydrate diet. A Mediterranean diet (containing olive oil, vegetables, low amounts of saturated fat, cereals, brown rice) is beneficial and, compared to a high fat Western diet, lowers the risk of having a heart attack.

> *The combination of lifestyle changes – being on a low fat diet, stopping smoking, exercising every day, managing and reducing stress, having good–quality, restful sleep and being generally happy, is very effective in relieving angina and reducing the risk of heart attacks.*

PRESCRIPTION PILLS

There are several groups and they work in different ways and are often used together.

Aspirin (over-the-counter)

This makes it less likely for platelet blood cells to stick together and this allows the "thinner" blood to flow more easily down the arteries. Aspirin, in a dose of 75 mg a day, is given to patients with all types of cardiovascular disease. It reduces the risk of death by 25% in patients who have coronary heart disease. All patients with coronary heart disease or any vascular disease (narrowing in any artery) should take aspirin unless they cannot tolerate it or if they have a very unusual allergy to it.

Clopidogrel (Plavix)

This is a newer and more expensive drug that works in a different way to aspirin but has the same effect in making the blood less sticky and so less likely to clot. It is no more effective than aspirin and the risk of bleeding from the stomach is similar. It is used in patients who cannot take aspirin and also in people who have had angioplasty and a stent.

Beta Blockers

These are the pills ending in "-ol." Most are taken once a day, but some need to be taken two or three times a day. They are several different types with slightly different actions, but they are similar.

Some beta blockers are combined with other drugs, like water pills or a calcium tablet, as a combined, single pill for the treatment of high blood pressure.

These are often used as the first treatment for angina and they are generally effective. They are also used to treat high blood pressure, heart failure, and heart rhythm problems and are given to patients after a heart attack. They are also used to treat migraines.

Angina occurs when the heart beats faster and more strongly, requiring more oxygen. Because beta blockers slow the heart rate and reduce the force of the contraction of the heart, they are a logical and effective treatment for angina.

The common side effects are: cold hands and feet (and so are generally avoided in people with peripheral vascular disease), depression, bad dreams, sluggishness of thought and ability to do things (this is why they are sometimes used to calm people down), impotence and dizzy spells.

They should not be given to patients who have a slow or abnormal conduction of electrical impulses down their heart (heart block), bronchitis and asthma or a very weak heart muscle. These side effects can be too much for some people and so around 30% of people cannot tolerate them and stop taking them (sometimes without telling their doctor).

Nitrates

Glyceryl trinitrate was first used for angina in 1867 and remains very good treatment. It acts almost immediately but is effective for only a few minutes. It should be taken before doing anything (walking fast, strenuous housework) that brings on the chest symptoms of angina. It is usually taken as a spray under the tongue but is also available as a very small tablet. It must be chewed or sucked because if it is swallowed, it is rendered ineffective by the acidic stomach juices.

The most common side effect is a headache. Some people take too much within a short period of time, which can lower their blood pressure so much that they faint. This is called a "nitrate faint." Some patients don't like taking it because of the headache it produces.

Long-acting Nitrates (eg, isosorbide)

These are effective and useful in some patients and are given to try to prevent attacks of angina. The problem with them is that a lot of patients may get "nitrate-tolerant" so that the drug loses its effect.

They should not be given to patients who take sildenafil (Viagra) because the blood pressure may fall.

The short-acting nitrate, glyceryl trinitrate, is very useful. Patients should take it before they do anything that they think might bring on an angina attack (walking, gardening). The side effects include dizziness due to a low blood pressure, weakness, flushing, and headache.

Calcium Channel Blockers

There are three main types. Heart muscle cells and blood vessels need calcium to work and contract. Without calcium, they do not contract as hard and this means they use less oxygen. All three calcium channel blockers block the entry of calcium into the cells of heart muscle and blood vessels. Calcium is also needed by the electrical heart muscle cells. A deficiency of calcium leads to a slow heart rate.

1. Verapamil
   Used mainly to treat high blood pressure, it can cause low blood pressure with dizziness, slowing of electrical impulses in the heart and a very slow heart rate, constipation and headache and flushing.
2. Nifedipine and amlodipine
   These are used to treat high blood pressure and angina, often in combination with a beta blocker because they produce a fast heart rate that is counteracted by the beta blocker. They relax and widen the arteries of the heart and the legs, causing a lower blood pressure. This allows more blood to get to the heart muscle.
   The common side effects are of flushing (red face), headache, swollen feet, and palpitations.
3. Diltiazem
   This is a very useful drug to treat angina and high blood pressure. It slows the heart and should not be used in patients with a slow heart rate. It can be given once or more a day. Side effects are uncommon but include flushing, dizziness, and low blood pressure and slow heart rate in high doses.

Nicorandil

This is, at present, one of a kind. It increases the amount of potassium in cells. It is usually used in combination with other types of drugs to treat angina. Side effects include headache and flushing.

WHICH TYPE OF DRUG IS THE BEST?

No group of drugs is "better" than another in treating angina. Beta blockers, despite their common side effects, are useful in patients after heart attacks because they have been shown to reduce the risk of future heart attacks whereas the other angina drugs do not.

OTHER DRUGS USED IN PATIENTS WITH ANGINA

Statins are used in patients with angina, even those who have a "normal" cholesterol level, because they make the fatty plaques stable and less likely to rupture. They are also useful in patients with unstable angina for the same reason. Statins in big doses slow the progression, and in some patients reverse, coronary heart disease. The target LDL-cholesterol level in patients with angina or unstable angina or previous heart attack is less than 2.0 mmol/l.

Statins also reduce the inflammation in arteries.

ACE Inhibitors

Angiotensin converting enzyme inhibitors should be given to patients with angina if they also have high blood pressure, diabetes, previous heart attack, and a weak left heart pumping chamber (left ventricle) and to those with kidney problems but who can tolerate an ACE inhibitor.

WHY DON'T WE DO CORONARY ANGIOGRAMS IN ALL PATIENTS WHO MAY HAVE CORONARY HEART DISEASE?

Coronary angiography carries a risk of heart attack, stroke (in around 1 in 1000), and death (1 in 1000). The test may cause other problems, for example, bruising or damage to the artery in the leg. Some people are allergic to the contrast fluid we inject.

They are also exposed to X-rays. Some patients find it painful or uncomfortable. Patients need to take the day off work. Coronary angiograms are usually done by cardiologists and can be done only in certain hospitals by doctors with the necessary training.

CORONARY ANGIOPLASTY: WHAT IS IT AND WHAT HAPPENS?

This procedure, first performed by a radiologist in Switzerland, has revolutionized the treatment of coronary heart disease. It is used in all types of patients, of all ages. It is used to treat patients with a heart attack, as well as those with angina, who previously would have needed heart bypass. It is quicker and less expensive than a bypass. It doesn't have the same risks as a bypass. The risks of death are similar. Most patients would prefer to have angioplasty.

The new stainless steel meshes (stents) reduce the risk of the artery blocking off and the results are as good as surgery.

Angioplasty is now done as an emergency treatment for patients who are having or who have had a recent heart attack. It has been shown to be more effective in opening up a blocked heart artery than clot-busting drugs (thrombolytics). The risks of angioplasty in treating heart attacks is slightly higher than in treating angina.

SO WHY DO HEART BYPASS SURGERY AT ALL?

Angioplasty is done whenever technically possible. Surgery is used when angioplasty is not possible (the arteries are not suitable). Heart bypass surgery is a big operation but still, for the right patients, a good and effective way of treating angina.

How Many Stents Can Be Put in?

Several. The number is limited only by space in the artery.

What Happens to the Stent?

It stays in the artery and becomes part of the heart artery wall. It becomes coated with the patient's cells within a month. After this time, the risk of a clot forming in the stent is much less.

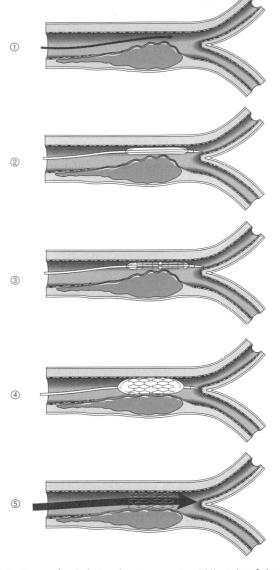

Figure 3.4: Diagram of angioplasty and stenting procedure. (1) Narrowing of a heart artery with fat. (2) The inside of the artery is opened or widened by inflating or blowing up a balloon at the end of a tube (angioplasty catheter). (3) The angioplasty balloon is removed. Another similar balloon or angioplasty catheter that has a steel mesh tube (stent) on it is positioned, as before, using x-rays, at the place where the artery is narrowed. (4) The balloon is blown up. The stent expands and remains expanded in the inside wall of the heart artery. The balloon is deflated and removed. (5) The stent, usually covered with a drug that reduces the chances of the artery narrowing down again, remains in the artery. Within a month, the stent is covered with the patient's cells.

Can the Stent Move or Fall Out?

Not after it has been fully expanded in the artery.

Are Stents Dangerous, and Can They Cause Heart Problems or Cancer?

No. The only problem, which is very unusual, is that clot can form in the steel stent before it becomes fully covered with the patient's own cells, which grow naturally around it. It is not yet clear whether drug eluting stents can cause some types of cancer.

Sometimes special drugs are given to patients who may have or are likely to develop blood clots in their arteries.

Can I Go through the X-ray Machine at Airports if I Have a Stent?

Yes.

Can I Go into an MRI Scanner?

Yes.

WHAT PILLS ARE RECOMMENDED AFTER ANGIOPLASTY?

Aspirin and any other pills your cardiologist thinks helpful. These may include a statin for the cholesterol, a beta blocker, an ACE inhibitor, or an Angiotensin II blocker.

WHAT PILLS ARE NECESSARY AFTER A STENT?

Nearly all patients who have angioplasty also have a stent implanted. Currently, a pill called clopidogrel (Plavix) is given for a year after the procedure. Drugs used to treat angina are usually stopped soon after the angioplasty.

WHEN CAN I GO BACK TO WORK AND DRIVE AFTER ANGIOPLASTY?

After one week.

WHAT ABOUT SEX?

As soon as the groin is comfortable.

WHAT ARE THE CHANCES THAT I WILL NEED ANOTHER ANGIOPLASTY?

There is a 10% risk that the treated artery will narrow down again even if you had a stent put in. Because the new drug-coated stents have not been around for long, it is difficult to be sure how long the artery will stay open.

Patients who do everything they should do to keep their arteries open, do much better than those patients who do not.

Arteries are more likely to narrow again after angioplasty in patients who have high cholesterol, who continue to smoke, who are diabetics, who have kidney disease or high blood pressure, and any other risk factor.

WHY DO PEOPLE GET ANGINA AFTER ANGIOPLASTY?

Around 10% of patients treated with angioplasty may get angina again within a year if the artery that has been treated narrows again. We now use "drug eluting stents" which leak drugs into the wall of the heart artery. These drugs reduce the chances of the artery narrowing again (*restenosis*). These relatively new drug eluting stents, when used with other drugs to lower cholesterol, and to reduce the risk of blood clotting, have reduced the restenosis rate to around 5%.

If angina occurs more than one year after angioplasty, it is more likely to be due to a narrowing in a different artery or at a different place in the same artery.

An exercise test is helpful and then a coronary angiogram is usually done to see precisely what the cause of the angina is. Whether the artery has narrowed in the same area or a different artery has narrowed, angioplasty can be used again.

HOW MANY TIMES CAN ANGIOPLASTY BE DONE?

Several. But every time it is done, there is a slightly increased risk of damage to the leg artery or whichever artery is used to gain access to the arterial system. Sometimes the wrist or radial artery is used.

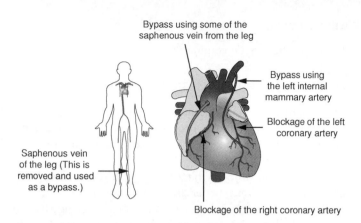

Bypass using some of the saphenous vein from the leg

Bypass using the left internal mammary artery

Blockage of the left coronary artery

Saphenous vein of the leg (This is removed and used as a bypass.)

Blockage of the right coronary artery

Figure 3.5: Heart bypass: The left internal mammary artery is a branch of the artery to the left arm (the left subclavian artery). It is freed from the inner chest wall and then inserted into the left coronary artery, past the blockage.

CORONARY ARTERY BYPASS SURGERY

What Is a Bypass?

This is a big operation and is being refined. The principle is the same. Whereas angioplasty opens up a narrowed or blocked artery, coronary artery surgery bypasses the blockage. A vein or artery is used as the connection tube. The tube carries fresh blood containing oxygen from the heart, bypassing the blockage, and inserts into the normal part of the heart artery. This allows fresh blood to get to the heart muscle.

Why Is It Done?

To improve the blood supply to the heart muscle in patients with angina.

Can It Be Done to People of Any Age?

Yes, although the risks are higher in the elderly, because they are more likely to have other things wrong with them, for example, kidney problems and a tendency to stroke, because their neck and brain arteries are likely to be narrowed.

WHAT ARE THE RISKS OF HEART BYPASS SURGERY?

Depending on the patient, around 2% risk of death. In some, it may be higher, particularly the elderly if they are having other heart procedures, for example, a valve replacement too. The risks are higher in patients who have had a heart attack within two months; this is why the operation should be postponed if possible. A freshly damaged heart muscle is soft and electrically irritable and may tear and go into dangerous rhythms. The risk of heart bypass increases in older patients, those with lung, kidney, or liver damage. The risks of stroke are higher in the elderly and in those who have narrowing in their neck or brain arteries, or who have fat deposits in their aorta, or a calcified, hard aorta.

The veins are taken from the lower part of the legs, usually the left leg. This may occasionally cause an infection in the skin. The leg from where the vein is taken usually has a tendency to be slightly swollen.

Most surgeons still cut the breastbone with an electric saw. Occasionally, the breastbone does not knit together, which can give problems and pain. If the breastbone does not knit together, then another operation to fix it may be necessary.

There is a risk of stroke and loss of memory after the bypass. Usually this is not severe and most patients recover completely. Most people are able to get back to full activities and end up fitter and have a healthier lifestyle after their bypass.

What Should Be Done before the Operation?

Get as physically and emotionally fit as possible:

- Stop smoking.
- Get your blood pressure checked.
- Make sure your lungs and your arms and legs are strong.
- Have a healthy diet.
- Get your blood sugar and cholesterol checked and take treatment if necessary.
- Get slim.
- Speak to the nurses and support groups before the operation so that there are no surprises.

HOW DO I KNOW THAT I NEED THE OPERATION?

Heart bypass operations are done to treat angina. If you are in doubt about having it, speak to your cardiologist and/or heart surgeon if you have any doubts. Usually, angioplasty would have been considered first. Heart surgery is offered to patients when the cardiologist considers angioplasty a less effective or safe option, or technically not possible. Also, heart surgery is often considered a more effective treatment if the heart muscle is weak and if the main left artery is narrowed.

DO BOTH ANGIOPLASTY AND HEART SURGERY MAKE YOU LIVE LONGER?

Both angioplasty and coronary artery surgery are done primarily to relieve angina when pills and lifestyle changes have not worked.

Although angioplasty improves angina and allows more blood to get to the heart muscle, it has not been shown to increase life expectancy.

Heart bypass surgery, however, improves life expectancy but only in patients who have a severely weakened heart muscle and important narrowings in all three heart arteries, or if the origin of the left artery (which gives rise to the two main left arteries) is severely narrowed.

WHAT TESTS ARE DONE BEFORE I GO INTO THE HOSPITAL FOR A HEART BYPASS?

Blood tests and blood typing, chest X-ray and ECG. If your have bad breathing, lung function tests may be necessary.

WHO DOES THE OPERATION?

The heart surgeon and his team. There is also an anaesthetist, a perfusionist (a technician who makes sure that your body gets enough blood and oxygen during the operation), nurses and other operating room staff.

CAN I HAVE THE OPERATION AT ANY HOSPITAL?

No. Only one where heart surgery is done.

HOW LONG DOES THE OPERATION LAST?

Around three hours. It takes time to put you to sleep, "harvest the vein," put you on "bypass" (making sure that when the heart is stopped in order to sew the grafts on, there is blood getting around your body), cutting open the breastbone and exposing the heart and the blocked arteries, and then the bypass grafts have to be connected to the aorta and the heart arteries.

OFF PUMP BYPASS: WHAT IS IT?

This is a newer way of doing the operation. It is not done by all surgeons and is also not suitable for all patients. The patient is not put on a bypass machine and the heart is not stopped. The grafts are sewn on to the heart while it is still beating. This is technically more difficult and special equipment is used to stabilize the heart as much as possible. It does not permit such easy, controlled access to all parts of the heart. "Off pump, beating heart" surgery may carry a lower risk of stroke (the aorta, which may have lots of fatty deposits, is not clamped), the patient does not have the risks of surviving on the bypass machine, which may contribute to the brain and psychological problems after bypass, and the smaller incision in the chest means that there is less pain for the patient after the operation and the patient can get up and about more quickly. They may be able to leave hospital after a few days, and recovery is quicker and less painful.

Not all patients need to go to the intensive care unit after the operation. Antibiotics and painkillers are given, a urinary catheter in used until patients can go to the toilet easily, and they are given physiotherapy and encouraged to get out of bed very soon after the operation and encouraged to walk.

WHEN CAN BYPASS PATIENTS RESUME FULL ACTIVITIES?

As soon as they can, increasing the amount they do every day. Depending on the type of work they do, they should be able to go back to work, part time initially, after 6–8 weeks.

They will be encouraged to walk as much as they can, increasing the distance if they feel able. They should get into the habit of eating a healthy diet, having a rest or nap after lunch, taking their pills on time, and getting to bed early for the first month.

They should not drive for at least six weeks, but this, together with their return to work, depends on their particular case (what was done and how it was done), and the views of the surgeon and the team at the hospital. Things have changed a lot recently, and patients are made to feel more relaxed, positive and encouraged to get back to normal earlier than before.

WHAT PILLS ARE NEEDED AFTER BYPASS?

This depends on your condition. Aspirin is generally recommended for life in everyone who can take it. All the cardiovascular risk factors have to be checked and treated if necessary. The really important things – smoking, blood pressure, weight, diet and exercise – have to be really well controlled in order to reduce the risks of further problems after the operation.

CARDIAC REHABILITATION

This should start before the operation. The hospital classes usually start a few weeks after the operation and patients find them reassuring, helpful, and fun and allow them to speak to other patients and share their experiences.

WOUNDS

These usually heal up quickly. If a wound looks infected or is painful or opens up, patients should contact their doctor.

When Is It Safe to Resume Sex?

When you and your partner are in the mood. The chest wound, particularly in patients who have had their breastbone cut, may be sore and tender for weeks and vigorous sex can displace the bone. You will have to think about this and may need to modify your position and technique. Until your confidence returns, don't expect things to be immediately as they were before the operation. Your partner may be more anxious than you and it is a good idea to discuss this with your doctor or the nurses in the rehabilitation unit if you have any concerns.

ALCOHOL

There are no rules about this. It is best not to drink for the first month after the operation. Many people find that they have lost their taste for alcohol for the first few weeks. You may find that you are more sensitive to alcohol and it is sensible to restrict it to one unit a day after the first month until you feel completely back to normal. Because it can irritate the heart rhythm, and is fattening, you should drink in moderation (less than 10 units per week) even after you have fully recovered.

DOES ANGINA RETURN LESS COMMONLY AFTER CORONARY ARTERY SURGERY COMPARED TO CORONARY ANGIOPLASTY?

Yes. Angina occurs less commonly and much longer after coronary artery surgery than after angioplasty. It is usually due to a narrowing in one of the bypass grafts but sometimes may be due to further narrowing of a heart artery that was only slightly narrowed, or normal, and therefore not bypassed at the time of the operation. Exercise testing and coronary angiography are usually done. Narrowings in grafts or one of the patient's own (native) arteries can often be treated with angioplasty and stenting at the time, or shortly after the angiogram.

SO SHOULD PATIENTS HAVE ANGIOPLASTY OR BYPASS SURGERY? WHICH IS BETTER?

It isn't a matter of which is the better treatment. Both techniques are designed to improve the blood supply to the heart and to reduce the amount of angina a patient has.

> *Usually angioplasty is recommended if the cardiologist who is going to do the angioplasty thinks that all the arteries could be treated effectively and safely.*

Bypass surgery may be recommended:

- If the arteries have been completely blocked for a long time (more than one year, which makes it unlikely that the artery can be opened).
- If the arteries are very tortuous (it is technically more difficult and more risky to try to pass the balloon and stent through arteries that are "curly- wurly", because the arteries may get torn (dissected).
- If the arteries are very calcified. Arteries containing a lot of calcium may not be suitable for angioplasty because it may not be possible to open them up with the balloon.
- If the arteries are narrowed all the way down. This makes it less likely that angioplasty will be successful. Opening up the top of the artery may not improve the flow of blood further down if the artery is severely narrowed downstream.
- If the patient also needs a heart valve replacement.
- If the patient has a very weak heart muscle. Patients with a very weak heart muscle are at high risk of death in any event, whether they take pills or whether they have angioplasty or surgery. Surgery has been shown in one big trial to reduce the risk of death in patients who have a very weak heart muscle and in whom all three main heart arteries are narrowed.
- When previous angioplasties have not been successful.
- When the patient definitely prefers bypass surgery.

WHAT ARE THE DOWNSIDES OF HEART BYPASS SURGERY?

It is a big operation. Depending on the patient, his age, the state of his heart, whether he has kidney damage, liver damage, bad lungs (most commonly due to previous smoking damage), a previous stroke or a risk of stroke, bad circulation in his leg arteries, the risk varies between 2–10%. In most low-risk patients, the risk of death during or shortly after bypass is around 2%.

IS THERE EVER A SITUATION WHERE BOTH ANGIOPLASTY AND BYPASS SURGERY ARE DONE TOGETHER?

Yes. Some cardiologists call this a *hybrid* or *combined operation*. The artery or arteries that are suitable for angioplasty are opened up with a balloon and a stent is implanted in the artery. The artery or arteries that are not suitable for angioplasty are treated with coronary artery surgery.

IS BYPASS EVER DONE WHEN ONLY ONE ARTERY IS AFFECTED?

Yes. If the patient has bad angina that does not respond to medication, and if angioplasty cannot be done safely or would not be thought to offer the patient relief from angina, then very occasionally, a heart bypass may be recommended.

Heart Attacks

Read this chapter to learn:

- that a heart attack is death of heart muscle cells resulting from a blood clot blocking off a heart artery
- that the typical symptoms are chest pain, breathlessness, and sweating
- 50% of victims die suddenly, without warning
- what to do if you think you are having a heart attack
- what treatment is given and what tests are done
- what problems can occur after a heart attack
- how to get back to a normal life and what patients should do to do to live longer
- what problems can occur in patients who have had a heart attack.

WHAT IS A HEART ATTACK?

A *heart attack* is death and damage to the heart muscle. This is caused by a blood clot in one of the three main heart arteries, blocking the supply of blood to the heart muscle.

The clot in the heart artery blocks the supply of blood, oxygen, and nutrients to the heart muscle. Without blood and oxygen, the heart muscle cells die within one hour. Unless the blood supply to the heart muscle is restored within one hour, the muscle cells will not recover. Some recovery of some of the cells may occur if their blood supply is restored within six hours. After 12 hours, the cells cannot recover. This is the reason why it is crucial for patients with heart attacks or suspected heart attacks to phone for an emergency ambulance so that the diagnosis can be confirmed and the condition treated immediately.

Patients with heart attacks are now being taken directly to the cardiac catheter laboratory for angiography to see if a heart artery is blocked and where it is blocked. The cardiologist will then decide what the best treatment is for the patient. This is often

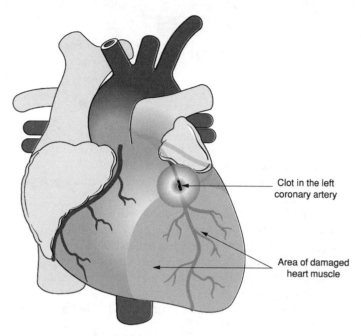

Clot in the left coronary artery

Area of damaged heart muscle

Figure 4.1: Heart attack: The clot in the heart artery blocks the supply of blood, oxygen, and nutrients to the heart muscle. The closer the blockage to the beginning of the heart artery, the more heart muscle is affected, and the more damage occurs. The greater the amount of heart muscle damaged, the greater the risk of death, heart failure, and disability.

angioplasty and stenting. The artery is opened with a balloon and a stent inserted into the artery at the site of the blockage. Drugs are also given to reduce the chance of further blood clots and all risk factors have to be treated effectively.

The closer the blockage is to the top (origin) of the heart artery, the more heart muscle is at risk of damage. The more muscle damaged, the greater the risk of death, heart failure and disability.

Sudden death, due to a fatal heart rhythm abnormality, may occur even when there is little muscle damage. This is why it is not helpful to describe heart attacks as big or small or major or minor. All heart attacks are potentially fatal. However, the more muscle damaged, the greater the probability that the patient will develop heart failure.

HEART ATTACKS ARE DUE TO CRACKING OF THE SURFACE OF A LAYER OF FAT (CHOLESTEROL)

Even a thin layer of fat (plaque) in a heart artery can cause big problems. The inside wall of the heart artery may get inflamed and the top surface of the layer of fat may crack. We call this a "ruptured plaque" of fat. Soft fat is more likely to lead to trouble than stable, hard fat. The soft fat consists mainly of the "bad" type of low density lipoprotein cholesterol, or LDL cholesterol.

The crack in the surface of the fat layer causes a blood clot to form at the site of the crack. The blood clot may, if big enough, and if not broken down or dissolved by the body's own clot dissolving mechanism, block off the artery completely. If no blood and oxygen get to the heart muscle cells, they die. This is called a heart attack.

WHAT ARE THE SYMPTOMS OF A HEART ATTACK?

- severe chest pain (pressure, heaviness, or a squeezing sensation)
- feeling short of breath
- sickness and vomiting
- collapsing and blacking out; 50% of people who black out never wake up.

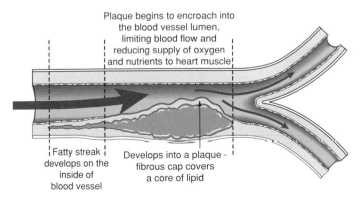

Plaque begins to encroach into the blood vessel lumen, limiting blood flow and reducing supply of oxygen and nutrients to heart muscle

Fatty streak develops on the inside of blood vessel

Develops into a plaque - fibrous cap covers a core of lipid

Figure 4.2: Stages of atherosclerosis.

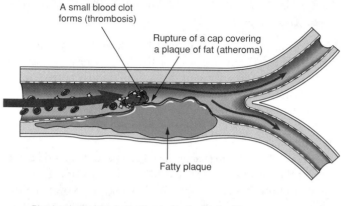

A small blood clot forms (thrombosis)

Rupture of a cap covering a plaque of fat (atheroma)

Fatty plaque

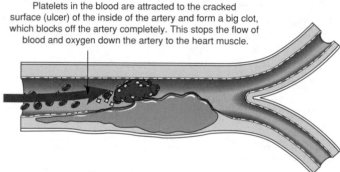

Platelets in the blood are attracted to the cracked surface (ulcer) of the inside of the artery and form a big clot, which blocks off the artery completely. This stops the flow of blood and oxygen down the artery to the heart muscle.

Figure 4.3: How heart attacks happen.

The symptoms of a heart attack last at least 20 minutes, and usually more than an hour. The pain in the chest may also be felt in the throat, jaws, and arms or only in these areas.

> *If you think you are having a heart attack, phone for an ambulance for immediate diagnosis and treatment. If necessary, you will be taken to the hospital.*

WHAT MAKES A PERSON LIKELY TO GET A HEART ATTACK?

Heart attacks are more common in older people and very uncommon in young people (under 40 years of age). They are more likely to occur in people who have angina and in those who have one or more cardiovascular risk factors.

WHAT CAN BRING ON A HEART ATTACK?

Anything that increases the amount of work the heart does, for example, exertion, sudden stress, and emotional upset and arguments can cause a heart attack. Sudden increases in the heart rate and blood pressure can cause layers of fat in a heart artery to crack. No obvious cause is found in most patients.

WHY IS CRACKING OF THE LAYER OF FAT IN THE ARTERY DANGEROUS?

Because blood clots form at the site of the cracked layer of fat, blocking off blood supply to the heart muscle.

DO HEART ATTACKS OCCUR WITHOUT WARNING?

Yes. Heart attacks occur out of the blue in people who have never had any chest pain and who were previously very fit and active, as well as in people who have had angina for a long time. Some people with stable angina notice that they get angina more frequently and it lasts longer. This is called unstable angina and can lead to a heart attack.

WHAT SHOULD PATIENTS DO IF THEY THINK THEIR ANGINA IS GETTING WORSE?

They should reduce their activities, and take plenty of GTN before they do anything that causes chest pain and also when they get chest pain.

If they are getting angina at rest or doing very little, they should go to the hospital for treatment.

CAN SOME PEOPLE HAVE A HEART ATTACK WITHOUT KNOWING IT?

Yes. Some heart attacks may be "silent," causing no symptoms at all. They may be recognized only when an ECG (electrical recording of the heart) is done for other reasons (check up or before an operation).

Silent heart attacks are more common in the elderly and in diabetics because they have a reduced sensitivity to pain.

IS HEART ATTACK PAIN JUST LIKE ANGINA?

It is more severe, lasts longer, and does not go away quickly after a spray of GTN. Patients with a heart attack may also feel sweaty and faint (they may lose consciousness); some feel as if they are going to die.

Although several conditions can mimic angina, fewer things mimic a heart attack. Some of these are equally dangerous and need to be investigated urgently.

HOW CAN YOU TELL IF A PERSON IS HAVING A BAD ANGINA ATTACK OR A HEART ATTACK?

It is difficult. It may mean having to go to the hospital for a blood test and ECG. Whereas angina would usually disappear after a few minutes, heart attack pain lasts for more than 30 minutes and it makes people feel very unwell.

WHY DO PEOPLE DIE FROM A HEART ATTACK?

The sudden lack of blood and oxygen to the heart makes the heart cells very irritable and this causes a serious rhythm abnormality. The heart stops pumping. Therefore, the circulation of blood around the body stops and no blood gets to the brain, the heart, the kidneys, and all the other organs of the body stop working. The organs of the body, from the brain to the toes, are starved of blood, oxygen, and nutrients, and the cells of the body die. The brain dies very quickly – within a minute or two – if it does not get any oxygen.

CAN DEATH OCCUR IF ONLY A SMALL PART OF THE HEART IS DAMAGED?

Yes. A cardiac arrest can occur even if only a few heart muscle cells have been damaged. Therefore, death within the first few hours does NOT depend on how much heart muscle has been damaged but whether the damaged muscle cells are electrically irritable.

WHAT ARE THE CHANCES OF SURVIVING A HEART ATTACK?

Thirty percent of people who have a heart attack die before reaching hospital. This is usually because the normal heart rhythm changes into an abnormal heart rhythm called ventricular fibrillation (sometimes called a "VF arrest"). Sometimes the heart just stops beating and there is no electricity in the heart muscle (called an "asystolic" = no heart action – cardiac arrest).

After 10 minutes, with the heart stopped, there is very little chance of restarting the heart, even if the patient had an arrest in the hospital. The longer the heart is in the abnormal rhythm, the less likely it is that the patient can be resuscitated (brought back to life), and the less likely that other organs of the body will be saved and able to function. So, the abnormal heart ventricular fibrillation rhythm (not to be confused with the common and usually harmless, atrial fibrillation), has to be converted back to normal within a minute or two.

Around 10% of patients who reach the hospital, die in the hospital. The risk of dying is greatest in the elderly, those who have had a lot of damage to their heart, and those with cardiovascular risk factors, or who get a chest infection, a clot in their lungs (pulmonary embolus), or have bad kidney function.

Young, fit people can have heart attacks but they generally do well afterwards.

WHAT IS THE TREATMENT FOR A CARDIAC ARREST?

If the patient's cardiac arrest is due to ventricular fibrillation and the patient is given an electrical shock (defibrillated) successfully within a minute or two of the heart stopping, then survival is possible. However, the chances of survival are slim in the elderly who often have other medical conditions, and if the heart rhythm is not converted back to normal quickly.

WHAT HAPPENS TO PEOPLE WHO HAVE A CARDIAC ARREST OUTSIDE THE HOSPITAL?

Most die because they collapse, lose consciousness, and their blood circulation stops. Even though some members of the public are aware of basic life support, most do not do it often enough to do it properly. Most of the public would not know what to do in such a frightening situation. Unless resuscitation is done properly, there is little point in trying it. The aim is to make sure that oxygen can get into the patient's lungs and to restore the circulation of blood around the body.

AREN'T THERE DEFIBRILLATORS IN SOME PUBLIC PLACES?

Yes. There are in some underground and railway stations, supermarkets, and airports. But unless they are used within a minute or so, by people who know what to do, they are of no use.

WHAT ABOUT MOUTH TO MOUTH RESUSCITATION?

If done properly, this can maintain life by blowing oxygen into the lungs. Pumping the chest must also be done to keep the circulation going until an ambulance arrives. If it is not done correctly, then it is unlikely to be of any benefit. Compressing the chest of an elderly patient is likely to fracture the ribs.

How Can Resuscitation Be Learned?

Contact the Red Cross or your local hospital for details.

IS THERE SUCH A THING AS A "BIG" OR A "SMALL" HEART ATTACK?

The terms are confusing and are not used nowadays because they are misleading. Big and small refer to the amount of heart muscle damaged, but it is very difficult to measure the size of a heart attack.

Ultrasound of the heart, blood tests, and a chest X-ray give an estimate of how much the heart has been damaged. People who have had a lot of heart muscle damage may be breathless and generally do worse than people who have had little damage to their heart muscle. Ventricular fibrillation (the deadly cardiac arrest rhythm) occurs in people even if there has not been a lot of heart muscle damage. So death can occur even if there has not been a lot of muscle damage.

People can live a surprisingly good quality of life despite having had quite a lot of damage to their heart muscle, while others can have quite troublesome angina having had only a little heart muscle damage.

WHAT ARE THE CHANCES OF LIVING A NORMAL LIFE AFTER A CARDIAC ARREST?

Good, if the patient had been previously well and had been quickly resuscitated.

SHOULD PATIENTS WHO HAVE HAD A CARDIAC ARREST SEE A SPECIALIST?

Yes. Patients should be seen by a cardiologist for an examination and tests, and then a decision can be made on the best treatment. This could be medication, an angioplasty, or a heart bypass operation. Occasionally, a device, like a pacemaker, which recognizes when the heart rhythm is abnormal, is used, but this depends on the results of tests.

> *For young people who have had little damage to their heart muscle and whose blood supply to their heart is good, the future is good, providing that they do everything necessary to reduce the chances of another heart attack.*

> *It is important that patients who may be having a heart attack call for emergency help. The paramedics have the necessary training to make a diagnosis, record an ECG, and give treatment, including clot busting drugs.*
>
> *The earlier treatment is given, and the sooner a blocked artery is opened, the better. The longer the delay in opening a blocked artery, the more muscle is damaged and the worse the outcome.*

WHAT HAPPENS IN THE AMBULANCE?

The paramedics will ask the patient about the symptoms, check pulse and blood pressure, and do an ECG. A very small tube (cannula) will be placed in a vein on the back of the hand or in a vein in the arm. This will allow the staff to give drugs for pain and a clot busting drug. Patients will be given aspirin as long as it has not recently given them a tummy problem, some oxygen through a mask, and a painkiller injection (diamorphine). Some ambulance crews will give a clot busting injection to try to open up the blocked artery.

WHAT HAPPENS AT THE HOSPITAL?

- Is the pain from the heart and, if so, is it a heart attack?
Once a blockage has occurred, the first hour is the most crucial. The most important thing to know is whether patients have had or are having a heart attack, when it occurred, and what should be done. The type of treatment depends on when the heart attack occurred. If it occurred more than 12 hours previously, there is little point in rushing to try to open the blocked artery with clot busting drugs or angioplasty, unless patients are still having angina or the ECG shows that the heart artery is unstable. This means that the heart artery is clotting off and then opening up on its own. The reasons for this are not known.

- In the Emergency Department
Patients are seen by a doctor or nurse to decide whether they may have had a heart attack. They are asked questions, examined, blood pressure and pulse taken, and heart rhythm checked on a monitor. The amount of oxygen in their blood will be monitored with probe clipped on a finger. They will be given an oxygen mask to increase the amount of oxygen getting to their heart. An electrical recording of their heart (ECG), blood tests, and possibly a chest X-ray will be done.

- Does a normal ECG exclude a heart attack?
No. Only around one-third of patients who have had a heart attack have typical changes of a heart attack on their ECG. Most may have some minor abnormalities and this can make treatment difficult. The complete changes may take a day or more to develop. This is why it is often not easy to be sure that a patient has had a heart attack when they first come to the hospital and why the ECG has to be repeated.

- Heart enzyme tests
Heart enzymes leak into the blood from damaged or dead heart muscle cells. The higher the level of the enzyme, the more heart muscle has been damaged. The chemical that is measured in the blood is called Troponin. It has to be measured 12 hours after the time the pain started. A low level is good and means

that it is very unlikely that the person has had a heart attack and it also means that the patient is at low risk from a heart attack in the near future.

If the doctors think that the pain is unlikely to be due to the heart, and if the ECG is normal, then the patient, particularly if there are no risk factors for coronary heart disease, can be reassured and can go home.

If the Troponin level is high, it is probable but not definite, that the patient has a problem with the blood supply to the heart and may have had a heart attack.

The Troponin level in the blood is high in people who have had a heart attack. The Troponin blood test, if high, is very useful in identifying patients at high risk who may need to stay in the hospital for tests and treatment. If the Troponin level is low, it identifies people at low risk from a heart attack and who may be sent home.

- What treatment is given?

Treatment for heart conditions change fairly quickly in the light of research. Currently the treatment is, depending on the patient:

- Oxygen to increase the amount of oxygen in the blood to help the heart muscle and all parts of the body.
- Diamorphine, a strong painkiller, is injected to relieve the pain and reduce anxiety.
- Aspirin to reduce the stickiness of the blood clotting cells (platelets) to reduce the chances of further blood clots.
- Clot busting drugs (thrombolytics, thrombus = clot, lysis = to break up). There are several types. They are now given as a quick (bolus) injection. In order to get the best effect, they should be given within 12 hours, and ideally within one hour, of the artery blocking off. This is estimated from the time the patient first experienced chest pain. They should not be given to patients who have had recent surgery, bleeding, trauma, who may have a tear in their aorta (aortic dissection) as the cause of their chest pain; recent stroke, tummy ulcers, uncontrolled high blood pressure. There is a 1% risk of stroke.
- Heparin, a blood thinner, is also given with the clot buster and continued for 24 hours.
- Nitrate injections for pain and to reduce the pressure in the lungs.

- Beta blockers – drugs which end in "-ol" – reduce the amount of work done by the heart by slowing the heart rate and lowering the blood pressure. They are used to treat angina and high blood pressure and heart failure.
- ACE inhibitors – drugs which end in "-pril" – also reduce the amount of strain on the heart. They are also used to treat high blood pressure, diabetes, and weak heart muscle.
- Statins – drugs which end in "-statin" – lower the cholesterol but also have other beneficial effects in arteries and may reduce inflammation in arteries.
- In some hospitals, if the there is a cardiac catheter laboratory (heart X-ray room) with the necessary staff and doctors able to perform the procedure, patients may be taken from the ambulance or the Emergency Room, directly for coronary angiography (X-ray of the heart arteries) and possibly coronary angioplasty and stenting.

WHO IS ADMITTED TO THE HOSPITAL?

Those who have had a heart attack (confirmed from their symptoms and the ECG) and those who have angina that is threatening to turn into a heart attack.

Patients who are not well and in whom the cause of their problem is not clear may also be advised to stay in the hospital for tests.

HOW IS THE BLOCKED HEART ARTERY OPENED?

- A blocked heart artery may open on its own, without treatment (spontaneous opening) in around 50% of cases, particularly in young people).
- Clot busting drugs injected into a vein (given in the ambulance or in the hospital).
- Angioplasty and stenting in the hospital.

HOW CAN YOU TELL IF AN ARTERY IS BLOCKED?

Although the ECG is helpful, an X-ray of the heart arteries (coronary angiography) is the only way to find out if heart arteries are blocked. But it is not necessary to do this test in all patients, and the test can cause problems and complications in around 1 in

1000 patients. These include stroke, heart attack, and tearing (dissection) of the heart artery. Patients who have already been treated with clot busting drugs may get severe bruising in the groin after the angiogram and angioplasty because of continued bleeding, which is difficult to stop after the clot busting injection.

HOW QUICKLY SHOULD A BLOCKED HEART ARTERY BE OPENED?

Ideally, immediately. The quicker the blood supply is restored to the heart, the less damage there will be to the heart and the lower the chance of heart failure.

4

If the artery can be opened within one hour after the time when the chest pain started, most damage is prevented. More and more heart muscle cells die the longer the heart artery is blocked. There is very little point in trying to open a heart artery that has been blocked for more than 12 hours, unless the patient is still getting chest pain and the ECG changes suggest that the artery has not completely and permanently blocked off.

In most hospitals, where angioplasty cannot be performed, clot busting drugs are injected within 30 minutes of arrival. Aspirin, other medications, and injections are also given.

WHERE IS ANGIOPLASTY DONE?

Only in hospitals with a cardiac catheter laboratory, and with a team of cardiologists who are trained to do it.

IS ANGIOPLASTY BETTER THAN CLOT BUSTERS?

Angioplasty has advantages. Arteries are more likely to remain open for longer and there is a lower risk of stroke. But there are also risks in around 4% of patients and the artery can be damaged and there may occasionally be damage to the groin artery. Angiography allows a precise diagnosis to be made and also allows effective treatment. With angioplasty, the blocked artery can be opened up. It also allows the cause of the clot – the narrowed artery and the cracked plaque of fat – to be treated with a stent. Opening up and stenting a blocked heart artery gives a better result than simply dissolving the blood clot. However, it is slightly more risky than using clot busters. It is more expensive and technically a more difficult procedure than injecting clot busting drugs into a vein.

Sometimes, both treatments are used. The clot busting drug is given as soon as possible (often by the ambulance staff at the patient's home, or in the hospital emergency room). Then, angioplasty may be done if the clot busting drug does not appear to have worked.

Angiography (X-rays of the heart arteries) is done at the same time and provides information about the heart arteries; are they normal (and they sometimes look normal)? Are they blocked or narrowed? Where in the artery are the narrowings or the blockage? What is the heart muscle like – is it badly damaged or not? Has a heart valve (the inflow or mitral valve may be damaged) been damaged and is now leaky? If the valve is very leaky, the patient may be breathless due to the lungs filling with fluid. The valve may need repairing or replacing.

If angioplasty can be done within an hour, then it is probably better than clot busters.

SOME PEOPLE ARE KEPT IN THE HOSPITAL FOR SEVERAL HOURS WITHOUT TREATMENT. WHY?

In the majority of patients who come into the hospital, it is not possible to be sure that a heart attack has definitely occurred. Their symptoms may not be typical; the ECG may not be definitely abnormal; the blood test used – Troponin – a substance leaked from damaged heart muscle cells into the blood stream – has to be measured 12 hours AFTER the beginning of chest discomfort.

IS IT POSSIBLE TO TELL WHICH PATIENTS ARE LIKELY TO BE OK AND WHO PROBABLY HAVE NOT HAD A HEART ATTACK?

Yes. Young people with no cardiovascular risk factors, with symptoms that are not typical of a heart attack, and whose ECG and blood tests are normal, are at low risk and can go home. Sometimes, they are advised to come back to the hospital for an exercise test.

HOW DO I KNOW IF THE CHEST PAIN IS DUE TO A HEART ATTACK AND NOT INDIGESTION OR SOMETHING ELSE?

It can be difficult to distinguish between a heart attack and indigestion because both cause a similar type of chest discomfort. This is because the heart and the gullet develop from similar cells and have a similar a nerve supply. In the same way that we know if a finger has been burned (even without looking) because the sensation from the finger is represented in a certain area of the brain, so the heart and gullet are also represented in the same area of the brain. The brain finds it difficult to distinguish whether pain is from the heart or the gullet. They both feel the same! That's why indigestion is often called "heartburn." Therefore, people who have indigestion may think they have had a heart attack, and people who have had a heart attack may believe (and naturally would prefer to believe) that they have only indigestion.

WHAT HAPPENS AFTER THE ANGIOPLASTY OR CLOT BUSTING TREATMENTS?

Most people who have had a heart attack respond to the treatments given and feel quite well by the next day.

Patients who have no complications and have adequate support at home can leave the hospital usually the day after angioplasty or clot busters. There is less chance of an artery blocking off again after angioplasty because a stent   a steel mesh – is implanted in the artery at the time. However, after clot busting drugs, there is a one in ten risk of the vessel blocking again within a couple of days.

WHAT ELSE IS DONE IN THE HOSPITAL AFTER TREATMENT?

The period in hospital after a heart attack is a very good time for patients to think carefully about their lifestyle and how they want to live their lives in the future. They are offered advice and support from various members of staff who want to help them reduce the risk of another heart attack.

Patients are discharged from hospital much quicker nowadays. Fifty years ago, patients were kept in bed for six weeks because it was believed that if they got up and did too much exercise before this, they may have the rare complication of rupture of the heart. In those days (1950s), there were very few drugs available to help patients and the cause of heart attacks was not known. It was originally thought that the clot was a consequence, not the cause, of the heart attack.

Because patients with uncomplicated heart attacks may leave the hospital within 24 or 48 hours of the attack, it is important that they are given clear information on how to reduce their chances of another attack.

All aspects of prevention are discussed.

People who have had a heart attack have coronary heart disease and are at greater risk of having another heart attack than people who have normal heart arteries. Treating and controlling risk factors is therefore particularly important and more effective in them.

The key things are:

- stop smoking completely. Even one cigarette a day is dangerous. Counseling and nicotine replacement therapy are offered.
- make sure cholesterol and the LDL-cholesterol levels are low using diet, exercise and statins; all three approaches are more effective than one alone. A relatively new drug called ezetimibe is sometimes added to a statin in patients whose cholesterol remains high despite the statin.
- beta-blockers will be given (unless the patient has asthma or bronchitis or poor blood circulation in the legs).
- aspirin is given to reduce the stickiness of blood cells; clopidogrel, a drug that has similar effects as aspirin, is given to patients after angioplasty and stenting and also to patients who have had clot busting drugs.
- ACE (angiotensin converting enzyme) inhibitors are given to reduce the work of the heart; they also have beneficial effects on narrowed arteries. If patients cannot tolerate ACE inhibitors because of a dry cough (this occurs in around 20% of patients), they are given Angiotensin II blockers which have similar effects but rarely cause a cough.
- patients will be advised to get plenty of regular, daily exercise.
- identify and reduce stress; everyone has stress, and too much is not good for the heart and the arteries.
- eat a low fat, low carbohydrate, low salt diet with plenty of fresh fruit and vegetables.

- drink alcohol in moderation (no more than one unit per day).
- do not drive for four weeks. If patients drive a bus or taxi, they will have to "pass" an exercise test off heart medicines before they can return to work.
- patients can resume sex as soon as they feel in the mood, assuming they have no chest discomfort or breathlessness when walking.

GETTING BACK TO NORMAL

- **Anxiety and loss of confidence**

  It is common and to be expected that patients will have lost self-confidence and will be anxious after a heart attack. Now that they know they have a "heart problem," they are likely to feel very vulnerable at home and worry about all sorts of chest pains. It is important that they feel able to contact their GP and the practice nurse for advice and reassurance. Gradually they will begin to recognize what is normal and what is not.
- **Exercise**

  > *Exercise is probably the most important and effective way to regain self-confidence and a positive attitude.*

  If patients are able to walk fast and go upstairs easily without chest discomfort or undue breathlessness, then they will feel confident and optimistic.

  Physical exercise reduces the risk of dying from another heart attack substantially. Many people who have a heart attack end up fitter than they were before the heart attack, because they get into the habit of daily exercise. This also makes them feel fit and well and helps them reach a healthy weight. It reduces the cholesterol level, reduces blood pressure, and helps control the blood glucose.

  Exercise is the key to getting back to a normal quality of life. Patients should aim to walk for at least 30 minutes every day, gradually increasing the distance walked in that time. Ideally they should cover a mile in 20 minutes, though joint problems or lung problems may mean a lower target is right for them. Getting hot, sweaty and a little breathless is usually perfectly safe. This is part of getting fit. Initially, increase activity gently and don't try to do too much too quickly.

Walking, stair climbing, gentle cycling, swimming, dancing, tennis, and housework are all good to increase stamina. Lifting, vacuuming, carrying shopping bags, and using light dumbbells and exercising all arm muscles will improve strength.

Remember to stretch all muscles gently before and after exercise.

If you get angina or very breathless, dizzy or nauseous, or have palpitations (fast heart beat), stop exercising and see your doctor.

Once patients can walk upstairs comfortably, they are physically ready to resume sexual relations.

- Diet

  Eat a healthy, low fat, low salt diet with plenty of fresh vegetables and fruit. Avoid fast food, take-out, chips, crackers, cake, dairy products (cheese, cream, butter), ready-prepared meals, sausages, and fatty or fried food. Try to eat cereals, fish and lean meat, chicken, and turkey.

ARE THERE ANY TRUTHS IN SUPER-FOODS BEING ESPECIALLY BENEFICIAL TO PATIENTS WHO HAVE HAD A HEART ATTACK OR WHO HAVE CORONARY HEART DISEASE?

No. There is no reliable evidence that any of the foods written about in the papers or magazines have any special benefits to people who have had a heart attack or who have coronary heart disease.

Nevertheless, it is intuitively better to eat fresh fruit than a hamburger. There is also no evidence that any vitamin or folic acid prevents heart attacks.

- Work

  Most people stay off work for around six weeks but this depends on the patient, what their condition is like and if they had any important complications and what type of work they do.

  Patients should return to work as soon as they feel able. If they have a heavy manual job, then it may be up to six weeks before they have regained enough strength to know whether they will be fit enough to go back to doing the same job, or whether a less physical job would be better.

Psychologically many people feel that they should take some time off work after a heart attack. This can be useful to allow them to adjust their priorities. But leaving it too long is not a good idea.

When there has been a lot of heart muscle damage and patients get breathless walking just a few yards on flat ground, then returning to work may not be a good option. Patients might need more tests or treatment.

THE VALUE OF REHABILITATION COURSES

Most hospitals offer cardiac rehabilitation courses. Although some people may feel that this is unnecessary, there is something for everyone in rehabilitation courses. Information on the nature of heart disease and heart attacks is supplied, as well as help and advice to give up smoking, control cholesterol, control blood pressure, and control diabetes, diet, and weight. All of these are very important to reduce the risk of further heart problems. Exercise classes are predominantly for those with more severe damage or those who were not fit before their heart attack. Exercise rehabilitation classes are of less benefit to people who are fit and who can exercise without being told to do so.

WHAT IS THE RISK OF HAVING ANOTHER HEART ATTACK?

The risk of another heart attack depends on the age of the patient, the state of their heart arteries, as well as all their cardiovascular risk factors.

Information about the likelihood of further heart attacks can be obtained in many different ways. The number of narrowings in the heart arteries (other than the one that caused the heart attack) gives a very good idea of the future threat. This is most accurately assessed with a coronary angiogram.

Scar tissue in the heart can be seen using ultrasound. The function of the heart and the ability of the heart arteries to deliver sufficient blood and oxygen to the muscle can be assessed with an exercise stress ECG. As a result of this test and exercise tests on a treadmill or bicycle, a coronary angiogram may be advised.

Patients who have had a heart attack are more likely to have another heart attack than people with a normal heart. Many patients enjoy a long and untroubled life after a heart attack. Some need further tests and replumbing of their heart using either angioplasty or bypass surgery. All patients should be on medication, but not everyone takes the same tablets.

COMPLICATIONS OF HEART ATTACKS

Not all heart attacks are simple and uncomplicated, allowing early discharge and a return to normal activities. Some complications are so severe that the patient is likely to die in hospital or within some months. Some complications make patients less able to lead an active and normal life. Other problems last only a short time, and although severe, resolve, leading to more or less a full recovery.

Here are Some Examples:

- **Heart rhythm disturbances:**
  The heart normally contracts (beats) approximately once per second. If the timer that controls the heart rate is involved in the damage, the heart can occasionally end up going far too slowly or far too quickly. Serious rhythm problems (the type that cause sudden death) are most likely within the first hour after a heart attack, but the threat that they may occur remains for the first 24 hours. This is why patients have their heart rhythm monitored continuously for the first 24 hours. If the heart is severely damaged, then the risk of further dangerous rhythms is high. Sometimes, a special type of pacemaker (an internal defibrillator) may be advised.

  Often it takes some weeks to know how well the heart will recover after a heart attack, so this decision is often not made during the hospital stay.
- **Angina:**
  Further angina can occur after a heart attack. This is because the blocked artery may partially unblock without treatment or after clot busting drugs dissolve the clot, leaving a narrowing due to fat in the artery.

  The blocked artery may also remain inflamed for several weeks after the heart attack. This causes further blood clots to form and these can cause another full-blown heart attack or just episodes of angina, which pass off without too much trouble. If angina remains a problem, further tests, including coronary angiography, may be done and angioplasty or heart surgery advised.

- **Heart failure:**
  This is a weakness of the heart muscle, when 40% of the muscle has been scarred and is no longer working properly. Some people get breathless and have swelling or puffiness of the ankles. Others have no symptoms, possibly because they lead a quiet life and don't do much exercise. Having heart failure is not as bad as it sounds and there are, like most things, varying degrees of it. It may be so mild that patients don't feel any restriction in their activities. Others, who may be elderly and have other medical problems, may be very breathless doing very little.

> *Whatever the severity of heart failure, there are now treatments, which mean that most patients can expect a reasonable quality of life, despite the diagnosis.*

- **Rarer complications:**

Inflammation of the Lining of the Heart (Pericarditis):

This may occur two to three days after a heart attack. It causes chest pain, which is sharper and varies with position – usually being worse when lying down. This usually settles with painkillers.

Leaking Mitral Valve:

A murmur (a sound heard with a stethoscope) is often the first evidence that a heart attack has caused one of the valves to allow some blood to leak backwards when the heart is pumping. Often this is of no significance, it simply reflects the general heart damage, but occasionally this can cause severe breathlessness, and the patient may need an operation to repair or replace the valve.

Developing a Hole in the Heart:

Sometimes the ventricular septum, the muscular partition wall separating the right and left pumping chambers, is damaged, causing a hole in the heart. This allows blood to flow from the left to the right side of the heart. This puts more strain on the right side of the heart; less blood enters the left side of the circulation. An opertion to close the hole may be necessary. This can be done with a special closure device put in from the groin, under local anaesthesia.

WE ARE LIVING LONGER WITH CORONARY HEART DISEASE AND AFTER HEART ATTACKS. WHY?

Because medical care and treatment have improved. We understand more about how these conditions develop and what things really work in reducing our risk of getting them. Fewer adults smoke due to anti-smoking publicity, smoking clinics, help lines and medications (although smoking among children, teenagers and the twenty-year-olds, particularly females, may be increasing).

There is an awareness and acceptance that healthy eating and exercise are beneficial; we know that thinner people live longer and are more likely to survive longer after a heart attack.

High blood pressure and high cholesterol levels are treated more effectively and more aggressively in everyone, particularly those with coronary heart disease.

ASPIRIN THINS THE BLOOD; I DON'T HAVE CORONARY HEART DISEASE BUT SHOULD I TAKE IT?

Aspirin prevents the clotting cells (platelets) from sticking together into clumps and blocking off arteries. Because aspirin can cause bleeding in the gut, we advise only those who have vascular disease (fat in their arteries), to take it.

Diabetics are advised to take aspirin even if they do not have fatty deposits in the arteries because they are much more likely to get arterial problems.

DON'T MISS OUT ON THE BENEFITS OF EARLY TREATMENT FOR A HEART ATTACK

It's Only Indigestion, I'll Sleep It off!

Many patients who have had a heart attack stay at home and do not see a doctor perhaps for several days or longer. They may think that they have had indigestion or not want to believe that something is wrong. They may have had chest pain in the middle of the night and did not want to upset their spouse or partner and hope that it will all go away in the morning.

The Pain Is Still There, I Better Go to the Hospital.

Others come to the hospital only after several hours because their pain gets worse and lasts too long for indigestion.

It is for these reasons that many patients who have had heart attacks do not receive the benefit of heart attack treatments in the early stage when their heart artery has blocked off and when it could be opened, so reducing the amount of heart muscle damage. The longer a heart artery is blocked, the more heart muscle is damaged and the more likely the patient will have a weakened heart. The sooner the heart artery is opened and the blood supply restored to the heart muscle, the better the patient will do because less damage is done to the heart. The most useful time is within one hour ("the golden hour").

APART FROM INDIGESTION, WHAT ARE THE OTHER CAUSES OF CHEST PAIN?

There are several:

- pain from the muscle or ribs of the chest wall (injury, or muscle strain)
- chest infection or pneumonia
- clot in the lung (pulmonary embolus)
- pain from the spine
- a tear in the main artery coming out of the heart (aortic dissection)
- inflammation of the lining membrane of the heart (pericarditis)
- shingles
- anxiety about your heart

WHAT HAPPENS IF PATIENTS DON'T GET TO THE HOSPITAL WITHIN ONE HOUR?

All is not lost. There is still a lot to be gained if patients get to hospital within 6 hours but they will not, theoretically, get the maximum benefits from early opening of their heart artery.

ARTERIES CAN UNBLOCK ON THEIR OWN, WITHOUT TREATMENT

Around 30% of all blocked arteries, particularly in younger patients, may open up on their own (spontaneous recanalization). This explains why some people who have had a heart attack are found to have "normal" arteries with no blockages. What probably happened is that these younger people had a ruptured plaque of fat, a blood clot formed in the artery, blocking it off and causing the heart attack. Their own clot busting system (special chemicals circulating in the blood), or the clot busting drug they got in the ambulance or in the hospital, opened the artery up.

BLOOD CLOTTING AND CLOT BUSTING

We all have blood cells called platelets, which form a blood clot. For example, when we cut ourselves, we need platelets and the clotting chemicals to stop the bleeding. We also have a clot dissolving system, which works to break up blood clots when necessary. Unless there is a reason why they can't take it, we give all patients with narrowed arteries (cardiovascular disease) aspirin, most commonly in a dose of 75 mg (81 mg in the USA) every day to be taken with food. Some people can't tolerate it or it affects their stomach. There are other types of pills we sometimes use for these patients. The aspirin stops the platelets clumping together to form a clot. Because aspirin can cause bleeding from the stomach, we do not recommend it to everyone. Only those who have had a heart attack, a heart bypass or angioplasty, a stroke, angina or poor circulation in the legs and feet. Diabetics are given it because they are at risk of getting cardiovascular disease.

TESTS DONE AFTER A HEART ATTACK

- **Exercise test**
  Some patients may have an exercise ECG test. This is useful for several reasons. Patients who do well, are able to exercise for several minutes without chest discomfort, and who do not get any changes in their ECG are at low risk from a further heart attack. Patients who don't do well and get abnormal heart rhythms and changes in their ECG may need further tests including, perhaps, a coronary angiogram.

An exercise test done before patients leave the hospital is very reassuring to the patient, the family, and the medical and nursing staff. It saves the patient the anxiety of doing his own unsupervised exercise test when he goes home.

The main danger of a heart attack is damage to the heart muscle. We can get a lot of information about the heart muscle and how badly it may have been damaged with a simple clinical examination when the patient comes into the hospital. For example, if the patient has a fast heart rate, low blood pressure, and fluid in their lungs due to a weak heart muscle, this usually means that there has been a lot of heart muscle damage.

- **Chest X-ray**
  This is usually done when patients are admitted to the hospital. It is done to see if there is any fluid in the lungs due to heart failure.
- **Heart ultrasound (echocardiogram)**
  This harmless and painless test is very useful in seeing whether the heart is beating strongly or not.

> *There is a lot that patients can and should do for themselves to reduce their chances of having another heart attack.*

FACING THE FUTURE

Most people can get back to a normal life after a heart attack. Life has, however, changed. The risk of a further heart attack is higher once you have coronary disease, but it may be as little as 2–3% per year. Looking at this the other way around, there is more than a 97% chance that nothing bad will happen in a year. With such good odds, patients really need to get on with life.

For others, however, things are not quite so good. If patients have been left with a damaged heart and get breathless going up stairs, then they almost certainly need additional medicines for the heart and may have to adjust to a different pace of life. In addition, people who have been left breathless by a heart attack are more likely to end up in the hospital again. These days most people who have heart attacks are assessed during the first hospital admission to find out if further heart attacks are likely or not, and advised to have surgery or a stent if the risk is high.

Cholesterol and Other Blood Fats

Read this chapter to learn that:

- Cholesterol is the main fat (lipid) in the blood. It blocks arteries, causing angina and heart attacks. It is the most important and powerful cardiovascular risk factor.
- A high cholesterol level also increases the risk of having a stroke (lack of blood supply and oxygen to the brain, causing paralysis of one side of the body and sometimes loss of speech).
- The higher the cholesterol level, the higher the risk of coronary heart disease.
- The lower the cholesterol, the better, and the lower the risk of getting coronary heart disease and clogging in the brain and leg arteries.
- There are two types of cholesterol: the "bad" LDL cholesterol, which causes fatty deposits in the arteries, and the "good" HDL cholesterol, which protects against fatty deposits.
- Most people in the UK and US have high cholesterol.
- People who have high cholesterol plus one or more other cardiovascular risk factors (smoking, having high blood pressure, being overweight, being stressed, having diabetes or a close family member who had coronary heart disease under 60 years of age), are at much greater risk than people who have only a high cholesterol level. The more risk factors a person has, the greater their risk of having coronary heart disease and heart attacks.
- A high cholesterol level is most commonly due to a combination of eating a high fat diet and not taking enough exercise. Less commonly, it is due to a genetic problem.
- Thin people can have a high cholesterol level, and fat people may occasionally have a normal cholesterol level.
- Cholesterol is in dairy foods, eggs, fast foods (pizza, hamburgers, fried chicken, french fries, and chips), cakes, cookies, chocolate, animal fats, ready-prepared foods, liver, sausage, and many other foods.

- All types of alcohol increase cholesterol.
- "Low fat" labels on food are misleading. They contain more fat than you need or want.
- Avoiding fat, drinking very little alcohol (no more than one unit per day or preferably less), being slim and getting regular, daily vigorous exercise will lower the cholesterol by 10–20%. Doing all of these things is more effective than doing only one.
- People with normal heart arteries should have a cholesterol level less than 5 mmol/l, and the LDL cholesterol should be less than 3 mmol/l.
- The target level of cholesterol for people with clogging in any artery and in those who have had a heart attack or have had angioplasty or heart bypass surgery is less than 4.0 mmol/l, and the LDL cholesterol should be less than 2.0 mmol/l.
- Statins are a group of drugs that lower the cholesterol level by approximately 30%. They reduce the risk of heart attacks and stroke by 30%, and death by 20%. They are generally well tolerated and are more effective than diet in lowering the cholesterol level. Statins also reduce the likelihood of heart attacks and angina by reducing the inflammation in arteries and making the fatty deposits less dangerous.
- Statins are given to all people who have a blockage in any artery even if their cholesterol level is "normal" (<5.0). All patients who have had a heart attack, or have had angioplasty or heart bypass surgery, should be on a statin.
- Statins are also given to people with normal arteries if their risk of getting a heart attack or stroke is estimated to be more than 20% (based on charts). If a person with a high cholesterol is at low risk from getting a heart attack, she may not need a statin. Not all patients with high cholesterol need a statin.
- Other types of drugs lower cholesterol and other blood fats, which can be used with statins to lower the cholesterol and the triglycerides (another type of blood fat).
- There are no symptoms of high cholesterol. The only way to find out if your cholesterol is high is with a blood test.

WE NEED SOME CHOLESTEROL IN OUR BLOOD BUT NOT TOO MUCH

Angina and heart attacks (and stroke) are due to fat in the arteries. The blood fats are called *lipids*. There are several blood fats or lipids circulating in the blood. The main one causing blockages in the arteries is cholesterol. Although it causes problems when it gets deposited in the walls of the arteries, we cannot live without it. It has three main roles. It is an essential part of our cell walls, it is one of the chemicals used to make sex hormones (e.g., testosterone) and other steroid-containing hormones like cortisol, and it is also a component of bile acids, which are made in the liver and allow us to digest and absorb fats from the diet.

HOW IS CHOLESTEROL MEASURED?

Cholesterol is measured by a blood test. It can also be done with a finger prick test, which can be done in some pharmacies.

5

Should the Patient Fast before a Cholesterol Blood Test?

Although the total and HDL cholesterol levels are not significantly raised after a meal, the important LDL cholesterol and triglyceride levels are. Therefore, patients are usually asked to fast for 12 hours (but they can drink as much water as they like) before a blood test for cholesterol. Most patients find it most convenient to have their blood test in the morning. If the cholesterol level is high in a fasting patient, it cannot be due to a recent meal.

Cholesterol levels can vary a little in the same person from day to day.

APART FROM A BLOOD TEST, IS IT POSSIBLE TO TELL THAT A PERSON HAS HIGH CHOLESTEROL BY LOOKING AT HIM?

People with a high cholesterol may have deposits of cholesterol around the eyes (xanthelasma, pronounced zanthe lazmah), or around the elbow or over the back of the hands. Fat people often have a high cholesterol level. The only sure way to know if a person has high cholesterol is to measure the level in the blood.

CAN CHOLESTEROL BE TOO LOW?

No. The body makes all the cholesterol it needs even on a low fat diet. People with low cholesterol should be pleased. People with low cholesterol and low LDL cholesterol are at low risk from

---

angina and heart attacks, particularly if they do not have any other risk factors.

> **People who have had a heart attack, angioplasty, or bypass surgery should try to have cholesterol less than 4 mmol/l and LDL less than 2 mmol/l.**
>
> *The higher the level of cholesterol, the higher the risk of heart attack and death. A high cholesterol level is the single most powerful and dangerous risk factor for coronary heart disease. Half of all people who die from coronary heart disease have high cholesterol.*
>
> *The lower the cholesterol level, the better and the lower the risk of having a heart attack or stroke.*

IS HIGH CHOLESTEROL (AND OTHER RISK FACTORS) OFTEN DUE TO LIFESTYLE?

People with a high cholesterol level are often overweight because they eat too much fat and other unhealthy food, drink too much alcohol, and do little if any regular exercise. Because of all these factors, they often have or develop diabetes. Therefore, they have not only high cholesterol as a risk factor, but also, obesity, inactivity, and diabetes. If they also smoke, they are at particularly high risk.

All of these risk factors can be tackled with determination, hard work, and self-control.

BUT IT IS VERY DIFFICULT!

Yes it is. It depends on the person's attitude to their health and whether they want to increase their chances of living a longer and healthier life. People who have had a scare, for example, a heart attack, stroke, or a heart operation, often "wake up" and are able to make changes to their lifestyle.

CAN THIN PEOPLE WITH A HEALTHY LIFESTYLE HAVE HIGH CHOLESTEROL?

Yes. Some thin, active people who are very careful about their diet may have high cholesterol. This is due to a genetic problem in the way their body regulates and metabolizes cholesterol. If they have other risk factors, they may need treatment to lower their cholesterol level.

WHERE DOES CHOLESTEROL COME FROM?

Cholesterol comes from two sources. Most of it is made in the liver from the fats we eat, and we also get it from eating certain types of fatty food. There are two types of fat:

- the bad saturated fat (butter, cheese, and other dairy products, animal fat, drippings, lard, fatty meat, chocolate, cakes, cookies, pastries, chips, coconut oil). Certain "fast foods" (fried chicken, pizza, hamburgers, any food cooked in lard, butter, saturated oils), contain a lot of saturated fat. Saturated fat increases the bad LDL cholesterol.
- the less harmful, unsaturated fat (olive oil, soy oil, nuts, avocado, sunflower oil).

WHAT IS THE BEST WAY TO LOWER CHOLESTEROL?

The liver regulates the amount of cholesterol in the blood. The liver secretes cholesterol in the bile (which is stored in the gallbladder), which enters the gut. Therefore, there is a lot of cholesterol in the gut from the food we eat and the cholesterol made in the liver and then secreted into the gut. The most effective way to lower cholesterol is by both lowering the cholesterol made in the liver using a statin, and lowering the absorption of cholesterol from the gut into the bloodstream with ezetimibe.

ARE SOME FATS GOOD OR AT LEAST LESS HARMFUL THAN OTHERS?

Yes. Unsaturated fats are less harmful than saturated fats.

The more fat eaten, the higher the cholesterol level. The less fat eaten, the lower the level of cholesterol. All fats contain cholesterol, but some contain more cholesterol than others. It is better to eat unsaturated fat than saturated fat.

ARE THERE ANY OTHER GOOD FATS?

Yes. The oils in fatty fish, for example, herring, mackerel, sardines, kippers, salmon, trout, and tuna (particularly fresh tuna) contain good fats called omega-3 fats. We also make omega-3 fats from the oils in walnuts and soy. Omega-3 fats reduce blood stickiness, but it is not known how much we need to take. The general guidance is to eat oily fish at least twice a week.

Would Eating Oily Fish Cancel the Effects of Eating Bad Saturated Fats?

No. Even eating the amount of fish oil contained in a shoal of mackerel would not cancel the bad effects of a daily diet high in saturated fat (fast food and hamburgers).

Do Fish Oils Reduce the Risk of Getting Angina or Heart Attacks?

Possibly. But fish oils are better for you than animal fats (butter, lard, drippings).

APART FROM EATING TOO MUCH SATURATED FAT, WHAT OTHER FACTORS INCREASE THE CHOLESTEROL LEVEL?

- too much alcohol (three or more units per day)
- a very underactive thyroid gland
- severe kidney damage
- not doing regular exercise
- obesity
- familial hypercholesterolaemia (FH), which affects 1 in 500 people and causes very slow clearance of cholesterol from the blood into the liver. People with FH may have a cholesterol level of 8 mmol/l or more. There is a very rare form of FH where the cholesterol level is very high (more than 20 mmol/l), causing death from heart attacks in childhood.

IS CHOLESTEROL FATTENING?

Yes. Fat is the most fattening part of our diet. The most effective way to lose weight is to reduce the amount of fat as much as possible. If you cut out the fat, you will lose weight. Losing weight is also very helpful in reducing and controlling blood pressure. Cutting down on starchy food and alcohol is also a very effective way of losing weight and controlling diabetes in adults.

Is a High Cholesterol Level Always Due to Eating Too Much Fatty Food?

Usually, but not always. Cholesterol levels are higher in people who eat a lot of fatty food, get little exercise, and are overweight compared to those who are thin, drink little alcohol, and have a healthy, low fat diet.

ARE THERE OTHER BLOOD FATS THAT CAUSE HEART PROBLEMS?

Yes. The other main blood fats (which together are called lipids) are called *triglycerides*. These are not as important a cause of blocked arteries as cholesterol but are still important causes of angina and heart attacks. Triglyceride levels are high in people who drink a lot of alcohol, eat a lot of fatty food, or have diabetes.

WHAT ARE THE TWO TYPES OF CHOLESTEROL – THE "GOOD" AND THE "BAD"?

Cholesterol, being a fat, does not dissolve in water or blood. It is carried around the blood in "packets" called *lipoproteins*. There are two types of lipoproteins, which contain different amounts of protein (figure 5.1).

- Low density lipoprotein (LDL) "bad" cholesterol
- High density lipoprotein (HDL) cholesterol

The rest of the cholesterol is transported around the circulation in high density lipoprotein (HDL) packets. The HDL contains a lot of protein. This is the good, protective, cholesterol and reduces the amount of cholesterol in the arteries by taking it away from the arteries to the liver for excretion. Even if the total cholesterol is high, if nearly all of it is HDL cholesterol, then the person is still at relatively low risk compared to a person with a high LDL cholesterol.

Most (75%) of the cholesterol is carried around in the blood in the low density lipoprotein (LDL) "packet." It carries cholesterol from the liver to the cells. The cholesterol gets deposited

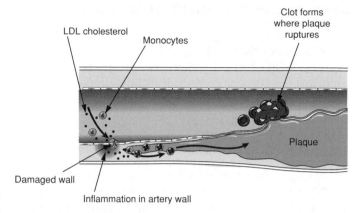

LDL cholesterol

Monocytes

Clot forms where plaque ruptures

Plaque

Damaged wall

Inflammation in artery wall

Figure 5.1: How cholesterol is deposited in arteries.

Cholesterol travels around the body in a packet made of protein called lipoprotein (fat protein). There are two types of cholesterol: low density lipoprotein (LDL) and high density lipoprotein (HDL).

LDL cholesterol travels from the liver to the arteries and gets deposited in layers called plaque. It is this LDL cholesterol that damages the arteries, causing a build-up of fat, which may crack, causing a heart attack or angina. It is referred to as the "bad" cholesterol.

The HDL cholesterol travels from the arteries to the liver and is protective, which is why it is referred to as the "good" cholesterol.

For various reasons, the lining of an artery may get inflamed. This damages the wall and allows LDL cholesterol to enter the inner wall of the artery. Layers of LDL cholesterol then get deposited in the inner wall of the artery, forming a bigger and bigger lump of fat. This causes a narrowing of the artery, reducing the blood flow to the heart.

The fat is soft and, under certain conditions, the cap or top surface of the fat may crack, or rupture. Even thin layers of fat may rupture, which is why young people can have heart attacks.

Medications that lower cholesterol ("statins") not only lower the amount of cholesterol in the blood but also firm up or "stabilize" the cap on fatty plaques, making them less likely to crack open.

in the walls of the arteries, causing blockages, angina, and heart attacks. It is called "low" density because it contains little protein. The higher the level of LDL cholesterol, the higher the risk of angina and heart attacks. The lower the LDL cholesterol level, the lower the risk of angina and heart attacks. It is very important for everyone to have a low LDL level and particularly important for those who have had a heart attack or have coronary heart disease.

WHAT IS A GOOD, SAFE LEVEL OF LDL CHOLESTEROL?

Everyone should have an LDL cholesterol less than 3 mmol/l and ideally less than 2.0 mmol/l.

WHAT ABOUT PEOPLE WHO HAVE CORONARY HEART DISEASE OR HAVE HAD A HEART ATTACK?

The LDL cholesterol should be even lower in people who have coronary heart disease (those who have had a heart attack or heart procedure); they should have an LDL cholesterol of less than 2.0 mmol/l.

> *The best and safest combination is to have low LDL cholesterol and high HDL cholesterol, and a low total cholesterol.*

What about the Ratio of Cholesterol to HDL Cholesterol?

This should be less than 4.5. The lower the ratio (total cholesterol level divided by the HDL level), the better and the lower the risk of coronary heart disease. A high ratio means that the HDL level is low, which indicates a higher risk of coronary heart disease.

HOW DOES THE CHOLESTEROL GET INTO THE WALL OF THE ARTERY?

The "bad" LDL cholesterol circulates in the blood and sticks to the wall of the arteries. Cholesterol is more likely to be "forced" into the wall of the artery in people with high blood pressure. The LDL cholesterol is taken up by the cells of the artery wall after it has been changed or "oxidized" by the addition of oxygen. This is why it was thought that foods and drugs containing antioxidants might reduce the amount of cholesterol in the artery. Unfortunately, none of these antioxidants, for example, vitamin E, has been shown to be helpful. Indeed, vitamin E may be harmful.

SO, SHOULD I STOP TAKING VITAMIN E?

Yes. If you have a healthy balanced diet, you do not need additional vitamin E. Any extra vitamin E you take is a waste of money and does not reduce your risk of getting coronary heart

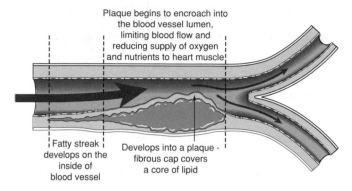

Plaque begins to encroach into the blood vessel lumen, limiting blood flow and reducing supply of oxygen and nutrients to heart muscle

Fatty streak develops on the inside of blood vessel

Develops into a plaque - fibrous cap covers a core of lipid

Figure 5.2: Stages of atherosclerosis

disease. But you should discuss this and any other changes with your doctor.

IS ATHEROMA THE SAME AS CHOLESTEROL?

The main constituent of atheroma is cholesterol. Plaques of cholesterol get deposited in the inside of arteries from a very early age. The arteries that are mainly affected are those in the brain, the neck, the heart, the aorta, and the leg.

Unless the cholesterol level and in particular, the LDL cholesterol, is lowered, more fatty material is deposited on top of the fatty plaque. This may obstruct the artery, resulting in angina. Plaques may become unstable. The surface may crack (rupture) and a blood clot form on top of the plaque, causing unstable angina or a heart attack and death.

IS CHOLESTEROL MORE LIKELY TO BE DEPOSITED IN ARTERIES IN PEOPLE WHO HAVE OTHER RISK FACTORS FOR CORONARY HEART DISEASE?

Yes. A high cholesterol level is even more dangerous in people who have any other risk factor. So a person with high cholesterol and any one or more of the following risk factors:

- smoking
- high blood pressure (hypertension)

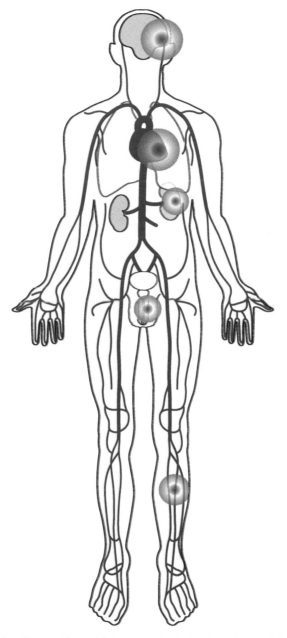

Figure 5.3: Diagram of the arterial circulation and main sites where atheroma (cholesterol) is deposited.

- diabetes
- overweight
- inactive
- family history of heart problems at a young age
- kidney problems

is very much more likely to get blocked arteries and have a higher risk of heart attack and stroke than someone who only has high cholesterol. The more risk factors a person has, the greater the chances of that person developing coronary heart disease and its consequences.

> *People with high cholesterol and any one of these cardiovascular risk factors will probably need medications to lower their cholesterol.*

WHAT CAN BE DONE TO REDUCE THE CHOLESTEROL LEVEL?

Eat less fat, particularly saturated fat. Having a very low fat diet and reducing alcohol can reduce the cholesterol and LDL level by approximately 10%. Alcohol does not contain cholesterol, but it interferes with the way the liver metabolizes it. If the cholesterol remains high despite these measures and the patient is doing their best, then medication may be necessary.

Exercise helps people lose weight, and people who exercise regularly usually control their diet, too. Exercise increases the "good," protective HDL cholesterol.

WHAT MEDICATION IS USED TO LOWER CHOLESTEROL?

The most commonly used and the most effective drugs are statins (they all end in "-statin"). There are five different types that all act in a similar way, although some are more powerful than others. They block the production of cholesterol in the liver by blocking an enzyme used in its production.

Simvastatin can now be bought over the counter in the UK. Statins are very helpful and effective drugs and have made a big difference to the way we prevent and treat people with coronary heart disease.

HOW EFFECTIVE ARE STATINS?

Statins reduce:

- heart attacks
- angina
- death from heart attacks
- strokes

Statins are now available combined with another medication called ezetimibe. Ezetimibe lowers cholesterol by reducing its absorption from the gut into the blood. This combination is even more effective than a statin alone but is more expensive and is used in people whose cholesterol remains high despite a big dose of statin. Combination drugs are more convenient for patients.

PRIMARY PREVENTION – TRYING TO PREVENT ARTERIAL BLOCKAGE IN SOMEONE WHO HAS NORMAL ARTERIES

A statin is used if a person is at an increased risk of getting vascular disease. This is estimated using special charts. These charts provide a very rough estimate of the probability that a person will have a heart attack or stroke within 10 years based on gender, age, blood pressure, cholesterol level, and whether or not they are a smoker and/or diabetic. A person's risk is lumped into risks of less than 15%, 15–30%, and more than 30% depending on which color section of the graph they fall into.

The charts are by no means perfect because they do not take into account other important risk factors (e.g., weight, level of activity, "stress levels," family history, and the number of cigarettes smoked). Also, the estimate derived from the table is very approximate and slightly misleading. A person who is estimated to have a 15% risk of having a stroke or a heart attack would be advised and prescribed a statin, but a person with only a slightly smaller risk of 14% may not be given a statin. The charts are only guidelines, not law. As in most areas of medicine, doctors use guidelines as guidelines and treat the patient in front of them because each patient is different.

Statins are also recommended for people with diabetes, even if they do not have vascular disease, because diabetics are very likely to develop vascular disease and are a high risk group.

Restricting statins to people estimated to have a risk of having a stroke or heart attack within 10 years, reduces the cost of treatment and targets those at higher risk. Using a risk cut-off value of 15% (in some countries the cut-off level used is 10%) means that people who may benefit from a statin may not be getting treatment that might reduce their risk of coronary heart disease.

In many countries, statins are available over the counter. It is important that they are taken only when there is a good reason and to remember that they do, occasionally, like all tablets, have side effects.

WHAT ABOUT THE USE OF STATINS IN PEOPLE WHO HAVE CORONARY HEART DISEASE (SECONDARY PREVENTION)?

- People with coronary heart disease – those who have had coronary artery surgery, angioplasty, or a heart attack, and those with angina should be on a statin.
- People with blockages in their leg (peripheral vascular disease) neck, or brain arteries, and those who have had a stroke or a "mini" stroke (transient ischaemic attack – cerebrovascular disease) should be taking a statin every day unless they cannot tolerate them, which is very rare.

Importantly, these patients should take a statin even if their cholesterol level is normal. The reason is that statins, whatever the cholesterol level, reduce the inflammation in arteries, and make the fat deposits in the arteries less liable to crack and cause trouble, for example, heart attacks and stroke.

> *People with furring up in any artery should be on a statin.*

WHAT ABOUT THE ELDERLY?

Statins should be used in the elderly although there is little information about their safety or benefits in people aged over 70 years. This applies to lots of other treatments in all areas of medicine because most drug trials exclude the elderly. The risks of drugs interacting with another, increase as the number of drugs taken, increases. Because elderly people are likely to have more than one medical condition, they are likely to be taking more than one drug. Therefore, they may not want to take another drug for a condition that does not worry them unduly, and if they do, they may get a side effect.

Some doctors may feel less inclined to prescribe a statin to elderly patients. Even though a 90-year-old is much more likely to have a heart attack or stroke than a 60-year-old, some 90-year-olds feel that they have managed to reach the age of 90 without statins, which may have side effects and make them feel unwell for the last part of their life, without making a significant difference to their lifespan. In these cases (as in all cases), the patient's views, assuming they are able to understand, should be taken into account.

SHOULD EVERYONE BE ON A STATIN?

No. The most sensible thing would be to discuss it with your doctor. Find out whether you should be on one or not depending on your risk factors (primary prevention) or whether you should be on one irrespective of your risk factors because of your medical history. They should not, like most other drugs, be used during pregnancy.

WHO SHOULD NOT BE ON A STATIN?

- People with liver disease
- People who drink a lot of alcohol
- People who cannot tolerate them

WHAT ARE THE SIDE EFFECTS OF STATINS?

Side effects are unusual. They include disturbance of liver function, painful muscles, gas, an upset tummy, and occasionally a rash. Very rarely, around 1 person in 100,000 may get a serious inflammation of the muscles in the legs and arms (rhabdomyolysis). This would get better over time when the drug is stopped.

How Do You Know if a Person Has Side Effects?

A blood test, to check the liver function, the cholesterol levels, and the muscle enzymes, is taken 6–8 weeks after starting the statin and, perhaps, every six months thereafter.

WHAT HAPPENS IF THE LIVER FUNCTION TESTS ARE ABNORMAL AFTER STARTING THE STATIN?

If the liver function tests are more than three times the upper limit of normal, and stay at this level, then the statin should be stopped. Sometimes, a different statin can be tried, but this may cause the same problem. The different statin should not be started until the liver function tests return to normal, which they usually do.

WHAT HAPPENS IF THE CHOLESTEROL LEVEL REMAINS HIGH AFTER STARTING THE STATIN?

The dose can be increased, but the patient will need another blood test to make sure the bigger dose has not upset the liver blood test. Another drug, called ezetimibe, can be added in.

DOES THE CHOLESTEROL DECREASE AS THE DOSE OF STATIN IS INCREASED?

Yes, but only slightly. Doubling the dose of statin does not further halve the cholesterol level. Doubling the statin dose results in a further 10% reduction in cholesterol.

WHAT HAPPENS IF A PATIENT WITH HIGH CHOLESTEROL CANNOT TOLERATE THE STATIN?

There are other drugs.

Ezetimibe is a relatively new drug that blocks the absorption of cholesterol in the gut. It is usually used together with a statin and lowers the cholesterol level by a further 15%. The combination of a high dose of statin and ezetimibe can lower the LDL cholesterol by as much as 50%. It can affect the liver, and the side effects are diarrhea, nausea, headache, tummy ache, and occasionally a rash. On its own, it is not as effective as statins. It is not given with fibrates.

Fibrates are a group of drugs that lower the triglyceride level. They have little effect on the LDL cholesterol. They can also be used with statins, but the risk of muscle inflammation (myositis) increases. They can also cause tummy upsets, kidney problems, and impotence.

Nicotinic acid has a moderate lowering effect on LDL cholesterol. It is not used very commonly. It is used with a statin to treat patients who have a high triglyceride level and a low HDL cholesterol level. It can increase the protective "good" HDL cholesterol by 30%. The side effects are flushing and liver problems.

Bile acid sequestrants lower the LDL cholesterol by 15% and increase the HDL cholesterol level. They are rarely used nowadays because patients find the side effects of constipation, bloating, nausea, and flatulence intolerable.

5

Food, Drink, and Weight

Read this chapter to learn that:

- Most people in the US and UK are overweight, and many are seriously obese. This is due to too much fat tissue. A flat tummy is ideal.
- Nearly everyone who is overweight eats and drinks too much. Very rarely is it due to a medical condition or a problem with the glands. It is not because they have "big bones."
- Being overweight or obese is an important risk factor for coronary heart disease.
- People who are overweight are also likely to have a high cholesterol level, diabetes, and high blood pressure. Compared to thin people, they are much more likely to get coronary heart disease and suffer from angina, heart attacks, heart failure, and strokes. They are also more likely to get aches and pains in their back, hips, and knees and find it difficult to exercise.
- Losing weight is often all that is necessary to avoid drugs for high blood pressure, high cholesterol, and high blood sugar (diabetes).
- Obese people are often depressed and may not enjoy life. They are often breathless. Losing weight and keeping it off increases their life expectancy and makes life more enjoyable.
- Being overweight or obese is not an excuse to take life easy, but a very important reason to exercise.
- Obesity has also been linked to some forms of cancer.
- Obesity often starts in childhood. Overweight, inactive children often become overweight, inactive adults. They usually have overweight parents. Therefore, getting into good eating habits during childhood is crucial.
- Obesity in old age is very rare because obese adults rarely reach old age.
- Obesity increases the risk of heart attack and death. It is as dangerous as having diabetes or high blood pressure or being a smoker.

- Exercise helps in losing weight, but people lose weight only by reducing the amount of calories they consume. The foods and drinks that are high in calories are the ones most people like, and most people know which foods they are.
- The best, most effective, and safest way to lose weight is by reducing the amount of food, particularly carbohydrates and fats and by reducing alcohol. All types of alcohol are fattening.
- Obese people often snore and stop breathing for periods when they sleep (sleep apnea). This is usually cured by losing weight.

WHAT IS OBESITY?

Obesity means having too much body fat. Being obese rather than overweight is only a matter of degree.

WHAT IS BODY MASS INDEX (BMI)?

Body mass index is used by doctors and nurses as a measure of obesity. It is calculated by dividing your weight in kilograms by your height in meters.

Normal: 18.5–24.9 kg/m^2
Overweight: 25–29.9 kg/m^2
Obese: more than 30 kg/m^2

For example, a man weighing 70 kgs (154 lbs) and who is 1.9 m tall would have a BMI of 19.4 kg/m^2 which is normal. A BMI over 25 increases the risk of death and heart problems. A BMI exceeding 30 is a serious medical condition.

ARE THERE SIMPLER WAYS TO KNOW IF A PERSON IS OVERWEIGHT?

Yes: by looking in the mirror without clothes on. Most people know if they are overweight. Everyone should have a fairly flat tummy and men should have a waist measurement of less than 36 inches.

WHAT ARE CALORIES?

A calorie is a unit of energy. We all need a certain amount of calories to live. Calories are like fuel for our body. The more active we are, the more calories we need. The less active we are, the less we need. Calories we do not use are deposited as fat under the skin. For example, an active man who is over 30 would need around 2000 calories per day. A small person who does little exercise may need only 1200 calories a day. It is possible for a person who does little exercise to exist on 800 calories.

WHAT ABOUT MINERALS AND VITAMINS?

We need various salts (sodium as found in table salt, but be careful because too much is bad and increases the blood pressure), calcium, and other trace metals. We need vitamins. People eating a full, balanced, healthy diet would have enough vitamins in the food they eat without needing extra vitamins.

WHAT IS A BALANCED DIET?

A balanced diet should contain just enough calories for the needs of each person, depending on size and activities. It should consist of the following components in the percentages of the total calories required:

Table 6.1: Components of a Healthy Diet

Carbohydrates	60%
Fat	less than 20% and less than 10% saturated fat
Protein	20%
Eat as little cholesterol as possible	
Salt	less than 2 grams per day
Alcohol	no more than 2 units (glasses) per day

Folic Acid and Homocysteine

Homocysteine is a chemical made in the body and is an essential ingredient in making parts of our cells. It was suggested over 30 years ago that too much homocysteine caused fat deposits in arteries (atheroma) and that in young people, too much homocysteine would appear in their blood and urine. Folic acid is a cheap vitamin given to pregnant women; it lowers the level of homocysteine. It was thought until recently that giving folic acid to reduce homocysteine levels would reduce the risk of coronary heart disease, reverse atheroma, or decrease the risk of death in patients who had had a heart attack. It did not. Folic acid does not reduce the risk of heart attacks or death from heart attacks. Indeed, it appears to make things worse. Folic acid may also increase the risk of a heart artery narrowing down after a stent has been inserted at the time of angioplasty.

This is a good example of how an attractive and simple idea has been proven to be incorrect. Many people are probably still taking folic acid in the belief that it is a harmless vitamin that might do them some good. Many people like taking herbal remedies or health foods for the same reason. Unless the active constituent in the food or herb is known and can be identified and the amount measured, and a proper trial conducted, it is impossible to know whether a food is beneficial or harmful. People who take folic acid in the belief that it is good for their heart should discuss this with their doctor.

TEN SIMPLE PRINCIPLES OF A HEALTHY, BALANCED DIET

1. Children over the age of two years should be taught by example that they should get into the habit of eating a low fat, low salt diet. Fat children become fat adults at risk of dying unnecessarily young from heart attacks. Encourage children to exercise every day. Educate them at a very young age not to eat fast food, junk food containing fat and salt, ice cream and other fattening foods, including candy and chocolate.

2. Without driving yourself crazy and becoming obsessed, be aware of what you eat. Remember that as long as you eat a healthy diet, you should never be hungry. Don't go on a diet. Just eat healthy food and lots of it. This is particularly important for people with coronary heart disease or vascular disease.

3. Eat as little fat, sugar, and salt as possible. Fat contains twice as many calories as protein or carbohydrates.

4. Don't reward yourself with creamy, fattening desserts or chocolate, cakes, and cookies because you have not eaten much during the day. If you are trying to lose weight and get fed up or bored, don't stray from your healthy habits; you will feel even more fed up. Eating the very occasional creamy dessert (perhaps once a month) is not dangerous.

5. Lean meat, fresh fish, beans, carbohydrates (pasta, bread, rice, in moderation), and fresh vegetables and fruit are good for you.

6. Take-out and fast food are bad and fattening. They contain a lot of fat and salt. It is difficult to know what goes into it, how it is cooked, or who cooks it. Eat it if you must, but if so, only very occasionally, perhaps once a month at most.

7. Don't drink more than two units of alcohol per day. It is fattening and makes you feel less energetic the next day. A small amount of alcohol (one unit per day) may offer benefits, but there is no convincing evidence that red wine is better than any other type of alcohol. Alcohol is fattening. In excess, apart from all the other problems it causes, it increases cholesterol, weakens the heart, and causes rhythm problems.

8. Processed, canned, packaged, and ready-to-eat meals contain preservatives and lots of fat and salt. Even the "lower calorie" or "lean" meals are fattening. "Diet" drinks make you feel less guilty but may contain calories or sugar.

9. Be aware of claims in the press, TV, radio, and diet books that a certain type of food (we have had unsubstantiated claims for oat bran, garlic, vitamin E, and lots of other foods) protects against heart problems and will make you live a long life as a beautiful person. Be wary also about fad diets, for example, a high fat, high protein diet to lose weight. They can be dangerous and should not be followed for long periods of time because they are unbalanced and unhealthy.

10. There is no clinical scientific evidence that food supplements, vitamins, and health food protect against heart disease. A person eating a full balanced diet does not need any supplements. Keep it simple. There are no "superfoods."

Table 6.2: Approximate Caloric Content of Foods

Food	Calories
Bread (1 slice)	80
Croissant	250
Cornflakes (1 bowl)	110
Swiss style muesli	220
Butter (1 tablespoon)	100
Cheese (1 oz)	100
Sugar (1 teaspoon)	15
Vegetables (4 oz portion)	
Green beans	20
Broccoli	15
Cabbage	20
Carrots	20
Boiled potatoes	125
Baked potatoes	104
Fried potatoes	240
New potatoes	75
Tomatoes	20
Lettuce	15
Mushrooms	18
Cucumbers	15
Yogurt	
Plain, carton	180
Regular, 8 oz.	180–220
Sugar-free, 8 oz.	120–150
Sugar-free, fat-free. 8 oz.	90–120
Salad dressing	
Regular salad dressing (2 oz)	200
Fat-free dressing (2 oz)	30–60
Mayonnaise (2 tablespoons)	200
Fruit	
Banana	80
Apple	60
Cranberries	14
Melon	100
Dried currants (4 oz)	250
Avocado	300
1 Egg	90
Rice (1 cup)	200
Sugar (teaspoon)	15

Table 6.2: (*Continued*)

Food	Calories
Fast food	
Quarter-pounder	430
Double whopper	1066
Fried fish	250
Fries	250
Hot dog	240
Fried chicken sandwich	450
Fried chicken wing	145
Whole pizza	1000
Alcohol	
Beer (1 bottle)	150
Gin and tonic	170
Shot of spirits	120
Glass of wine	100
Milk	
1 glass of whole	150
1 glass low fat (2%)	120
1 glass skim	80
Orange juice (4 oz)	50
1 sandwich with cheese	700
Soft drinks (1 glass)	
Water	0
Coca-cola	155
Milkshake	560
Ice cream (1 big scoop)	
Vanilla	140
Chocolate	300
Peanut butter (2 tablespoons)	200
Cake and baked goods	
1 slice cake	250
Chocolate bar	250
1 Danish pastry	250
1 jelly doughnut	200

Content of fats and oils	Saturated fat	Polyunsaturated fat
Butter	66	4
Corn oil	13	62
Margarine	17	37
Sunflower oil	10	70
Olive oil	15	10

6

CONCLUSIONS FROM THE TABLE ABOVE

- Fat is fattening, particularly fast food.
- Alcohol is fattening.
- Sweet things (baked goods, chocolate, cakes, and cookies) are fattening.

LOSING WEIGHT THE SENSIBLE WAY

- Everyone can lose weight.
- Imagine yourself thin, with a flat stomach, able to exercise, and do everything you want without getting breathless. Get into your mind the body shape you would like to have and could realistically achieve.
- Don't be in a rush. There's no need to rush.
- Think about what you eat. Eat less fat, and don't eat junk food.
- Eat slowly.
- Eat lots of low calorie food. If you eat meat, grill it.
- Don't eat sauces that are full of mayonnaise or creams.
- Cut out sweets, chocolate, chips, and other high-calorie snacks. It is better to have two small healthy lunches than snack during the day or when you get home hungry.
- Cut down or, if possible, cut out alcohol.
- Do some form of exercise, preferably cardiovascular (jogging, cycling, walking on a treadmill, using a cross-trainer) every day.

ALCOHOL AND THE HEART

It has been suspected for some time that alcohol might protect people from coronary heart disease. This was observed in the French, who eat quite a lot of fat but have less heart disease than people in other countries. This might be because they drink quite a lot of red wine. It is a popular belief that a small amount of any alcohol, not just red wine, reduces the risk of coronary heart disease.

But it is still not quite clear whether alcohol is good for the heart because it does not seem to work in animals fed alcohol.

SHOULD I START DRINKING RED WINE?

No. It is not a medicine. It is better not to drink at all.

DOES ALCOHOL "OPEN UP THE ARTERIES"?

No.

ARE THERE ANY GOOD THINGS ABOUT ALCOHOL?

No. It may make you feel more relaxed, but this is because it lowers your performance and your standards of behavior. It is a depressant and a sedative.

WHAT ARE THE BAD THINGS ABOUT ALCOHOL?

There is no doubt that too much alcohol is bad, leading to heart problems (rhythm problems, weakness of the heart, and an increase in the risk of coronary heart disease because alcohol increases the cholesterol level). Alcohol also damages the liver, the brain, and the nerves and makes people depressed, forgetful, impotent, and less able to function normally. Alcohol in moderation (one unit per day) might reduce the risk of heart attacks, but it does not reduce the risk of death.

SO HOW MUCH ALCOHOL IS SAFE FOR PEOPLE WITHOUT CORONARY HEART DISEASE?

Less than 14 units per week (two glasses of wine per day or a pint of beer).

WHAT ABOUT PEOPLE WITH HEART DISEASE?

The same. It is safe for people to drink a small amount (one to two units per day) after a heart attack, coronary angioplasty, or heart bypass.

DOES ALCOHOL INTERFERE WITH DRUGS?

Yes. Alcohol theoretically interferes with nearly all drugs because they are broken down in the liver. However, it is only potentially dangerous with the following:

- Antibiotics (metronidazole used for infections in the gut).

- Blood thinner (anticoagulants) warfarin. The blood may not clot, and an alcohol binge can lead to severe bleeding from the stomach.
- Antidepressants and alcohol can lead to drowsiness and loss of consciousness.

SO ARE ALL THE CLAIMS ABOUT ALCOHOL AND RED WINE BEING GOOD FOR THE HEART REALLY TRUE?

It might be, but the evidence is not that convincing. A small amount of alcohol—a glass of red or white wine per day – is harmless (except in people who should not take alcohol at all). It is sociable, pleasant, relaxing, and enjoyable. And so, like many other things in life taken in moderation, alcohol is safe and enjoyable but does not make you live longer.

7

Exercise and Rehabilitation

Read this chapter to learn that exercise:

- is good for you and your heart. The more you do, the better.
- prevents coronary heart disease.
- reduces the risk of death after a heart attack.
- lowers cholesterol.
- improves angina and heart failure.
- reduces the risk of getting diabetes and makes diabetes easier to control.
- when combined with a healthy diet, helps people lose weight.
- makes the blood less sticky, reducing the risk of heart attacks and strokes.
- makes us feel better, less stressed, more self-confident, and generally better, stronger, fitter, and brighter.

INTRODUCTION

Most people in the UK and US do not get enough exercise. Children are not exercising as much as their parents or grandparents did, and this is partly due to less emphasis placed on competitive sports in schools, today's sedentary, lazy lifestyle of watching TV and playing computer and video games, and less opportunities to participate in team sports.

Regular exercise can be inexpensive (e.g., walking) and has many health and cardiovascular benefits. It should be a part of daily activities for people of all ages. Even a single exercise session is better than none. As listed above, exercise has several benefits. Even gentle exercise, for example, walking fast for one hour every day, has been shown to reduce the risk of angina and heart attacks by one third.

> *Inactive people are twice as likely to get coronary heart disease and have a stroke compared to active people.*
>
> *Inactivity is as powerful a risk factor as smoking.*

EFFECTS OF EXERCISE ON RISK FACTORS FOR CORONARY HEART DISEASE

1. **Obesity**

   Exercise alone has a modest effect on weight loss. Most people can lose approximately 6-7 pounds over three months. Some people lose no weight or may even gain a few pounds, and think it is because "fat turns to muscle." This may cause some people not to do any exercise. This is incorrect. Most people who exercise for leisure (and who are not competitive athletes or weight lifters), and who do not eat or drink more, will get thinner, be more toned, and lose fat. Fat cannot become muscle. Muscle bulk may increase. So people who do a lot of cycling or running on a treadmill may notice that their leg muscles are stronger and may be a bit bigger.

   When combined with a low fat, low carbohydrate diet, most people can lose 15 pounds over a few months but need to continue the exercise and healthy eating habits.

   People who are disciplined enough to do regular, fairly strenuous exercise, usually are equally disciplined when it comes to eating and drinking and control their weight without any problems.

2. **High blood pressure**

   Regular physical activity helps prevent high blood pressure. It lowers elevated blood pressure, often enough to make drugs unnecessary.

   People who do little exercise have a 35% greater risk of developing high blood pressure compared to active people. Cardiovascular exercise (fast walking, running, cycling) is particularly helpful and effective.

3. **Diabetes**

   Exercise lowers blood glucose and makes it easier to control the blood sugar in diabetics. Exercise combined with weight loss prevents adult onset diabetes (not the type that affects children who need insulin).

4. **Smoking**

   Regular exercise makes it easier for people who want to stop smoking, stop successfully. It has to do with self-discipline and wanting to feel better and be healthier.

5. **Cholesterol**
Exercise increases the level of the "good" protective high density lipoprotein (HDL) cholesterol. A high level of HDL cholesterol reduces the risk of coronary heart disease. People who exercise regularly tend to be slim, fit, and careful about what and how much they eat, and so tend to have low total cholesterol levels.

6. **Thrombosis**
Exercise reduces the stickiness of blood, making it less likely to clot and cause a blockage in an artery.

Exercise reduces the risk of angina and heart attacks. These benefits apply to people of all ages.

7. **Psychological effects**
Exercise makes people feel and look better and fitter. It reduces stress and anxiety and is a great "stress buster." Feeling fit, strong, and mentally sharp makes it easier to cope with life's daily pressures, challenges, and irritations. Exercise relieves depression. People who exercise regularly should encourage others to follow their example.

Exercise, combined with a healthy diet, little or no alcohol, no smoking, and plenty of good-quality sleep, is an effective, safe, and inexpensive way of staying mentally and physically on top of things – cool, calm, collected, and completely in control.

---

8. **Training effects**
Regular training and exercise make muscles bigger and stronger, make the heart stronger, and make it pump slower and more efficiently.

If a person stops exercising for more than a few weeks, the benefits are lost quickly. The muscles weaken and the fitness level falls. This is why it is so important to maintain fitness and to exercise at least three times a week.

9. Although less is known about the beneficial effects of exercise on cancer, there is some evidence that it may help prevent some cancers.

IS EXERCISE EQUALLY BENEFICIAL TO MEN AND WOMEN?

Probably, yes, but it may be more effective in post-menopausal women, possibly because it improves the risk factors that exert more influence and are more dangerous to women after menopause. Exercise also has the added benefits in women of keeping their bones strong, which reduces the risk of osteoporosis (thin bones).

Walking at 3 mph for one hour each day has been shown to reduce the risk of heart problems in healthy women by at least 30% and overall in men and women by as much as 50%. More vigorous exercise provides even greater benefits.

HOW MUCH EXERCISE DO I NEED TO DO TO BENEFIT?

You should exercise enough to get sweaty and breathless. Thirty minutes every day would be enough. This should burn 1400 calories (the equivalent of a day's calorie intake in most people) per week.

Cycling hard for 20 minutes against a moderate resistance uses up 240 calories.

Is It Still Worth Exercising if I Can't Manage That Much?

Yes. Even a little is better than nothing. You can (and should) build up the amount you do.

HOW DO I START?

Just do it. Start walking fast, particularly if you see a hill or incline, and walk up stairs rather than taking the elevator. The best thing is to arrange your day so that you dedicate a fixed, regular slot for exercise. Going to the gym does not appeal to everyone. Having an exercise bike or treadmill at home (so that you can listen to music or watch TV to make it less boring) allows privacy, is cheap and convenient, and makes it easier for people to continue exercising during the wet, cold winter months. Use the cycle to exercise, not as a clothes horse!

Set yourself a realistic target. It is more important to do a little every day than a massive burn-out once a month.

> *The fundamental thing is to get into the habit of daily exercise, at a convenient time.*

If you do *not* have coronary heart disease or other medical problems, you could go to your local gym and get one of the trainers to help you with a regimen. Learn how to stretch before exercise, how to warm up, how and when to increase what you do, and how to cool down and stretch after exercise. These exercises help prevent straining your muscles and getting cramps.

BUT WHAT IF I HAVE A HEART PROBLEM?

If you have had a recent heart attack or get angina at rest or doing very little, do not start until you have seen your doctor, who may want you to see a cardiologist for further tests. If there is any suspicion that you may have a heart problem, for example, high blood pressure, see your doctor. Exercise is good treatment for high blood pressure, weak hearts (heart failure), and angina and is part of the treatment for people who have had a heart attack.

WHAT SORT OF EXERCISES ARE GOOD FOR ME?

Anything that makes you get hot, sweaty, and breathless. After exercise, you should feel relaxed and stress-free.

There are two types of exercise:

1. Stamina-type exercises that are good for the heart:
   (All these exercises should be started slowly and gradually increased. If you get any worrying symptoms, consult your doctor.)
   Walking fast, jogging, cycling, running on the road, track or treadmill, cross-training, playing tennis, swimming, dancing, doing vigorous housework, doing heavy gardening.
2. Straining-type exercises that are not so good for the heart:
   (These are not recommended for people with weak hearts or high blood pressure because they strain the heart and can put too much pressure on the heart muscle.)
   Weight lifting, rowing, exercising on machines to strengthen certain muscle groups.

WHAT ARE THE DANGER SIGNS TO LOOK OUT FOR DURING EXERCISE?

In people without coronary heart disease, the risks of exercise are negligible. It is more likely that you will pull a muscle than get a heart attack.

People with coronary heart disease should see their doctor if they get angina, undue breathlessness, dizziness, a feeling of their heart beating very fast or irregularly, or if they feel light-headed (which may occur if you do not cool down properly after vigorous exercise and just stop suddenly).

WHAT SPORTS OR ACTIVITIES ARE NOT HELPFUL TO THE HEART AND DO NOT REDUCE RISK FACTORS FOR CORONARY HEART DISEASE?

Darts, archery, tiddlywinks, fishing (except in a fast flowing river), and bowling (although there is some gentle walking involved).

Useful exercise has to involve a significant doubling of the resting heart rate, which is normally around 70 beats per minute.

BUT EXERCISE IS BORING AND UNPLEASANT!

Yes it can be, but you should always remember that it is very good for you and is a proven, effective way to help you to live a longer, more active, and less stressful life. Consider it as a treatment, like taking drugs, but often safer and more effective! Unless exercise is a bit unpleasant, you are not doing enough!

Exercising with a friend or a group of friends, for example, playing a sport together, jogging, going for a brisk walk, are ways to make exercise a pleasant and fun social activity.

It is very nice for parents to exercise with their children. It strengthens the relationship as well as getting children into good habits for life, which they can teach their children.

But It Takes Too Much Time out of My Day!

Whatever age we are and whatever we do during our day, most of us have 30 minutes that we can isolate for the good of our health. Taking time out for exercise will probably increase the time we have later!

I've Never Been Good at Sports, so How Can I Start Now?

Just do it. Everyone can and does improve the more they do.

How Can I Go to a Gym Looking the Way I Do?

Who cares? If you really are embarrassed, buy an exercise bike and exercise at home.

What if I Can't Afford a Cycle or a Gym Membership?

You can do a lot of useful exercise by walking up and downstairs, to the bus stop or the train station, or when you have time, in the park or even around the block after dinner.

Instead of watching TV, go for a walk.

But I'm Tired!

Exercise will make you more energetic and less tired; really!

IS IT SAFE FOR THE ELDERLY TO EXERCISE?

Exercise is even more helpful and important as we get older and helps us remain strong and independent. We should try to do more exercise every year. In this way, we are more likely to be able to walk, travel, go shopping, and look after ourselves.

Immobility and muscular weakness are two of the most common reasons why elderly people find it difficult to maintain social relationships and meet people. Social isolation is depressing and is a risk factor for coronary heart disease. Exercise allows elderly people to maintain social activities and remain socially active.

What Exercise Can the Elderly Do if They Are Not Very Mobile?

Elderly people can exercise the strength in their arms and legs while sitting in a chair by raising their legs for several seconds at a time. There are gentle, safe exercises they can do while lying down. Keeping the back and spine muscles strong and flexible is very important. Any movement is useful. They can get advice from their doctor or from a physical therapist. Some trainers have experience in advising the elderly how to remain supple and strong.

> *Keeping fit, active, and supple makes it more likely that you will enjoy a longer and more productive life.*

DOES EXERCISE REDUCE THE CHANCES OF DYING FROM A HEART ATTACK?

Yes. But you've got to do at least 30 minutes most days of the week.

WHAT IS "MODERATE" EXERCISE?

Walking briskly at 3 to 4 mph for long enough to get breathless. Slower but sustained walking may be adequate for elderly people. Carrying weights increases the work performed and the exercise intensity. Any exercise is better than none. A round of golf or walking the dog is only mild exercise, but better than sitting down, doing nothing.

Generally, irrespective of the fitness of the individual in question, exercise should result in a doubling of the resting heart rate for at least 30 minutes per day. Learn how to take your pulse instead of relying on the heart rate monitors on machines at the gym.

IS EXERCISE HELPFUL IN POST-MENOPAUSAL WOMEN?

Both walking and vigorous exercise reduce heart attacks and strokes in post-menopausal women regardless of race, ethnic group, age, and weight.

Vacuuming and making the beds are chores with health benefits!

WHAT ABOUT EXERCISE FOR THE ELDERLY AND PHYSICALLY LESS ABLE?

Although it may be impossible for elderly, bed-bound or chair-bound to exercise easily, they may nevertheless be able, with help and encouragement, to have passive exercise and breathing exercises. Elderly people can remain active and independent for longer if they are encouraged to remain physically and mentally active and supple, and to stretch their muscles.

Walking up stairs, even a few, is one of the simplest and most effective (and cheap) forms of exercise, and forces people to remain active. It's never too late to start, and being fitter and stronger makes it easier to enjoy life at any age.

IS EXERCISE EVER DANGEROUS?

Yes, but rarely in people who are generally active. If you have any concerns, consult your doctor. If a person is able to walk fairly fast on a flat slope without problems, then it is safe for them to do more. Some people, who have been inactive for years, can, to their surprise, increase their exercise capacity and strengthen up quite a bit.

Very occasionally, people who did not know that they had a rare heart condition die suddenly during vigorous exercise. This is usually due to an abnormal heart rhythm or the heart stopping. But bearing in mind how many people of all ages exercise, only a tiny number die as a result of exercising, and it is difficult to know how to prevent this sort of tragedy. People with a close family member who died at a young age during exercise should discuss this with their doctor; they may be referred to a cardiologist for assessment.

IS IT SAFE FOR PEOPLE WITH ANGINA OR A RECENT HEART ATTACK TO EXERCISE?

Yes, if they do not have angina at rest. Indeed, exercise is part of the treatment for these conditions.

IS IT IMPORTANT FOR CHILDREN TO EXERCISE?

Yes. This will reduce their risk of coronary heart disease because regular exercise reduces risk factors. It is very important for children and young people to get into an exercise habit for life.

Children need the practical example and encouragement of their parents and teachers and the time to do it. Parents should exercise with their children. Lots of sports can be done together, including jogging, cycling, playing tennis and soccer, and exercising in the gym

Competitive school sports should be seen as part of a step toward this life-long lifestyle. All children should be encouraged to do some form of cardiovascular exercise every day. Fit children are more likely to become fit adults.

> *Daily exercise is important for people of all ages, whether they have coronary heart disease or not. The more exercise taken, the better.*

CARDIAC REHABILITATION: EXERCISE AFTER HEART ATTACKS AND HEART OPERATIONS

Cardiac rehabilitation is a medical term for a range of exercise and education for patients with heart conditions, to help them regain their confidence, get them back on the road to an active and productive life, and lower their risk of having further heart problems.

Cardiac rehabilitation courses are run in hospitals for people recovering from heart attacks or who have had heart surgery. They should start almost as soon as a patient is admitted to the hospital at the time of the heart attack and before patients are admitted to the hospital for heart surgery or angioplasty.

Small groups of patients attend usually once a week and are taught about their condition, the risk factors for coronary heart disease, the treatments used, the tests done to investigate the condition, and ways to reduce the chances of getting another heart attack. A lot of time is spent teaching patients how to relax and cope with stress. It is very important that smokers stop permanently. Patients are taught to exercise and start a daily program of exercises that they should continue for life.

> *Rehabilitation reduces the risk of having a second heart attack by 29% and the risk of dying by 34%.*

WHAT ARE WAYS FOR PATIENTS TO GET THE MOST OUT OF A REHABILITATION PROGRAM?

Patients should be willing, motivated, and interested in prevention and the measures needed to improve their future. They should be prepared to use the 6- to 8-week program of two attendances per week as a springboard for continuing self-help healthcare and a lifelong commitment to regular exercise. Patients must take long-term, full-time control of their lives and be committed to a healthy lifestyle.

WHAT IS TAUGHT ON THE PROGRAM?

Patients are taught about how they can reduce their chances of another heart attack and what things work in slowing down the process of narrowing their arteries. They are encouraged to ask questions about their health, medical history, life stressors, and anxieties and may need a specialist's help for depression or psychological problems including personal, marital, or sexual problems. They are taught about their medication and why they should take it.

People who smoke or who drink too much alcohol, those who have been inactive, and those who have an unhealthy diet are given practical, straightforward advice on how to improve their lifestyle.

WHAT ARE THE RISKS OF DYING DURING CARDIAC REHABILITATION?

This is very rare indeed.

DOES EXERCISE HELP PATIENTS WITH BAD BLOOD SUPPLY TO THEIR LEGS?

Yes, very much so. Regular exercise triples the distance patients can walk. Exercise such as fast walking and cycling, particularly combined with other prevention, often dramatically improves the life of a patient with badly blocked leg arteries and claudication.

The greatest improvement is seen when patients are exercised to the point where the exercise hurts. This may create new channels and new blood vessels to carry blood to the leg muscles. Sometimes, exercise is as good as drugs and operations.

8

Diabetes

Read this chapter to learn that diabetes:

- is a blood sugar level greater than 7.1 mmol/l.
- is very common and becoming more common as people of all ages get fatter and do less exercise.
- is most common in adults between the ages of 60–75.
- increases the risk that a person will get coronary heart disease.
- increase the risk of death in patients with coronary heart disease.
- is the main cause of serious kidney disease requiring dialysis.
- in women is much more dangerous than it is in men; women are three times more vulnerable than men to the effects that diabetes has on the arteries. A diabetic woman is four times as likely to get coronary heart disease as a woman without diabetes.
- causes problems with several important arteries–the leg arteries (claudication), visual problems leading to blindness, kidney failure, numb feet, and weakness due to nerve damage and skin problems.
- results in 50% of diabetics dying within a year of their first heart attack; half of them die before they reach the hospital.
- increases the probability of needing heart bypass surgery and angioplasty.
- can result in patients going into coma if they are hungry.

HOW DO I KNOW IF I HAVE IT?

With a simple blood test. If your level of sugar (glucose) is high, you're a diabetic.

ARE THERE DIFFERENT TYPES OF DIABETES?

Yes. There are two types.

1. **Type 1** diabetes usually affects children and young adults who need to be treated with insulin. They notice thirst, weight loss,

and the frequent need to urinate. They need treatment with insulin for life because they do not produce enough themselves. They can sometimes go into a coma if their blood sugar falls very low or if the sugar level goes very high.

2. **Type 2** diabetes mainly affects adults who are usually overweight and do little exercise. It is uncommon for a fit, slim adult to get diabetes. Most patients with type 2 diabetes can be treated satisfactorily simply by losing weight and exercising every day. Some need drugs as well, and a minority need both drugs and insulin. In addition, women who have given birth to a baby weighing over 10 pounds is more likely to get type 2 diabetes later in life.

The aim of treatment for both types of diabetes is to regulate the blood sugar level very tightly within the normal range (3–6 mmol/l).

WHAT MAKES IT MORE LIKELY THAT A PERSON WILL DEVELOP DIABETES?

- Being overweight and inactive.
- Having a close family relative with diabetes.
- Being of South Asian/Afro-Carribean descent.

WHAT ARE THE MEDICAL PROBLEMS CAUSED BY DIABETES?

- Problems with large arteries causing coronary heart disease (angina and heart attacks), strokes, and claudication of the leg arteries, causing painful cramps when walking.
- Problems with small arteries causing blindness, loss of feeling in the hands and feet, impotence, and kidney disease.
- Skin problems, joint problems.
- High sugar levels can lead to a coma.

WHAT DRUGS SHOULD DIABETICS TAKE?

Some diabetics do not need drugs at all.

There are three different types of medication. Tablets are prescribed only if the patient fails to respond adequately to at least three months' restriction of carbohydrate and an increase in activity. The medications are aimed to augment the effect of diet and exercise, not to replace them. Patients who do not respond to diet and tablets may need to take insulin as well. The three main types of tablets used in type 2 diabetes are:

1. **Sulphonyureas.** They act by increasing insulin secretion. They can cause very low sugar levels (hypoglycaemia). Sulphonylureas are given to patients who are not overweight and in when patients cannot take metformin. Long acting suphonylureas are not often prescribed nowadays because of the risk of low blood sugars at night. Sulphonylureas may be combined with metformin or rosiglitazone.

   Patients may put on weight with sulphonylureas. They are not the drug of choice in the elderly and those with kidney impairment. The lowest possible dose should be used.

   Side effects are mild and include nausea and vomiting and tummy upset.

2. **Biguanides.** They work by decreasing glucose manufacture in the liver and increase the amount of glucose taken out of the blood into the cells. The only available one is metformin. It is useful in patients who are overweight and can be added to sulphonylureas, rosiglitazone or insulin.

   Side effects are unusual. It should not be used in patients with impaired kidney function.

3. **Other diabetic medication. Acarbose** delays the absorption of sugars from the gut. It is used with sulphonylureas or metformin. It cannot be given to patients with colitis. It may cause tummy upsets.

   Rosiglitazone increases glucose uptake into the cells from the blood. It can be used with other diabetic medications.

HOW IS DIABETES MORE DANGEROUS TO WOMEN?

Whereas type II diabetes increases the risk of coronary heart disease two-fold in men, it increases it three-fold in women.

Diabetes reduces the protective effect of the pre-menopausal state. So diabetics who still have periods are much more likely than nondiabetic women to develop coronary artery disease.

WHY IS DIABETES SO DANGEROUS?

A high level of sugar in the blood makes a person more likely to get blockages in the arteries and the layers of fat are more unstable; they crack open and get blocked by blood clots. High sugar levels make the blood sticky.

A high blood sugar level damages the kidneys, which leaks protein; this can be detected in the urine. People with kidneys that leak protein are 40 times more likely to die from a heart attack compared to people with normal kidneys.

The high sugar level affects all the arteries in the body, even the very small ones at the back of the eye. This can lead to cataracts and blindness. The small arteries that provide blood and nutrients to the nerves supplying the arms and legs may also be affected. This can cause weakness and numbness in the hands and feet.

> *It is very uncommon for a fit, slim, and active adult to get diabetes.*

WHAT ARE THE OTHER RISKS OF DIABETES?

Most diabetics are overweight and so are more likely to have high blood pressure and a high cholesterol level. Therefore, the single most important and effective way to control these important risk factors is for a person to be slim and active. They should also make sure that their blood pressure is "super low." Of course, they must not smoke. All of these important risk factors have to be controlled and treated, because a person's risk of getting coronary heart disease depends on the number of risk factors they have. The more risk factors, the greater the risk.

WHAT SHOULD DIABETICS DO ABOUT THIS?

They must see their GP and take their condition seriously. Although doctors can do tests, prescribe drugs, and encourage patients with diabetes, ultimately it is up to patients to do the things that will really make a difference to their lives. It may be difficult, but it will be worth it.

What Is "Super Low" Blood Pressure, and Is It Dangerous?

The blood pressure of patients *without* diabetes should be at or below 140/85 mm Hg. Diabetics are at greater risk of coronary heart disease. In order to reduce their risk, doctors, nurses, and the patients need to work even harder. The target for diabetics is

130/80 mm Hg – a lower level that is more difficult to achieve. Fifty percent of adult diabetics have high blood pressure. Controlling high blood pressure reduces the risk of kidney damage, stroke, and heart failure.

Drugs that are good for blood pressure and the kidneys (and also for the arteries and the heart muscle) are angiotensin converting enzyme inhibitors (ACE inhibitors), which are the drugs ending in "-pril". The angiotensin II antagonists, the tablets ending in "-tan", are also useful and are less likely to cause a cough.

SHOULD DIABETICS TAKE ASPIRIN EVEN IF THEY MIGHT HAVE NORMAL ARTERIES?

Yes. Diabetics are very likely to have, or to get, blockages in their arteries. They should take 75–81 mg of aspirin a day even if they do not have vascular disease. This is because aspirin makes the blood less sticky and less likely to form clots. Diabetics have sticky blood; they are advised to take it to reduce the risk of their already sticky blood, which could form a clot and block the arteries.

8

ARE THERE ANY OTHER DRUGS THAT DIABETICS SHOULD TAKE?

Yes. Diabetics, irrespective of their blood pressure, should take an angiotensin converting enzyme inhibitor (ACE). They should also take a statin even if their cholesterol level is low.

IS IT MORE IMPORTANT FOR DIABETICS TO STOP SMOKING THAN NONDIABETICS?

Yes. They halve their risk of having a heart attack within a year.

WHAT SHOULD DIABETICS DO ABOUT THEIR CHOLESTEROL?

Keep it very low. In all diabetics, the cholesterol should be less than 4.0 mmol/l, the LDL cholesterol should be less than 2.0 mmol/l, and the triglycerides should be less than 2.0 mmol/l.

Diabetics, even those who may not have coronary heart disease should take 75–81 mg of aspirin a day; they should also take a statin cholesterol lowering tablet in a big dose. If they have a high level of the blood fat triglyceride, they may need to take another drug called a fibrate, to lower their risk of coronary heart disease.

DO DIABETICS FACE ANY OTHER RISKS?

They are likely to get kidney problems. They should avoid non-steroidal anti-inflammatory drugs (for example ibuprofen).

Diabetics taking metformin should stop it for 24 hours before and after a coronary angiogram or other X–ray test using contrast fluid, which can damage their kidneys, particularly if they are dehydrated due to fasting before the test.

WHAT ABOUT ANGINA IN DIABETICS?

Even though diabetics are more likely to get blocked arteries, they are less likely to feel the consequences. They are less sensitive to angina, and this may explain why they may be too relaxed about their health because they do not feel anything–and this is the danger. People with symptoms or pain are more likely to look after themselves because they are aware that something is not right.

> *Diabetics don't feel the high blood sugar, the high blood pressure, or the high cholesterol level until. . . they have a heart attack.*

WHAT ABOUT HEART ATTACKS IN DIABETICS?

Male diabetics are 50% more likely to get a heart attack than nondiabetics; female diabetics are two and half times more likely. One third of diabetics die from a heart attack. So even though diabetics may not feel angina because they have a faulty warning system, they can assume that they have a one in three chance of dying from a heart attack. They should make sure that their blood sugar and their other risk factors are tightly controlled.

Diabetics who have heart attacks are more likely to die and sustain more heart muscle damage leading to more heart failure later. Once diabetics have a heart attack, they are at increased risk of further problems. The best way they can improve their chances is to follow the advice of the doctors looking after them.

ARE THERE PROBLEMS WITH ANGIOPLASTY OR HEART BYPASS SURGERY?

Yes. The narrowing process in arteries of patients with diabetes is different. The layers of fat material are less likely to be a single blob but more like a thick layer of fat spread all the way along the artery. This means the arteries look smaller and make these procedures technically more difficult and less successful.

Diabetics are more likely to get a complication or die after these procedures. For example, after bypass surgery, infection of the scars in the chest and legs is more common. Chest infections and kidney damage can also make things tricky and slow the recovery.

IS THERE ANY FOOD OR DRINK THAT DIABETICS SHOULD EAT OR NOT EAT?

They should cut out as much carbohydrates (bread, pasta, potatoes, sweet foods) as possible and eat a low fat, low salt, healthy diet with lots of vegetables. They should also avoid fruits containing a lot of sugar (mangos, lychees, and pineapple). They should not eat cakes, cookies, jams, chocolate, sweets, raisins, and other sweet foods. Even low sugar foods contain quite a lot of sugar.

Sweet drinks and soda full of sugar are bad. All types of alcohol contain sugar and are bad.

THAT DOESN'T LEAVE MUCH!

It leaves diabetics enough to enjoy themselves and live. But as long as things are done in moderation, it is not terrible to have the odd glass of wine, or piece of chocolate or sweet dessert or cake. It all depends on self-discipline and having the rare, planned treat rather than eating as much as you like and making excuses.

9

High Blood Pressure (Hypertension)

Read this chapter to learn that hypertension:

- does not make you feel ill, and only very rarely causes headache or nosebleeds.
- is NOT the same as feeling stressed, tense, or "hyper."
- is a pressure higher than 140/85 mm Hg in the arteries.
- is dangerous and increases the risk of getting coronary heart disease, angina, heart attacks, and strokes. It also causes heart failure by making the heart work harder and causes kidney damage and eye problems.
- affects 80% of people aged 70 and older and is equally common in men and women.
- runs in families.
- is more common in people who are overweight and who do little exercise. When they lose weight and exercise, their blood pressure may return to normal so that they can avoid taking drugs.
- is the second (after smoking), most preventable cause of death in the UK and the USA.
- is not controlled adequately in most people.
- usually needs treatment with at least two different types of drugs for life.
- can be monitored by patients using their own blood pressure machines.

WHAT IS HIGH BLOOD PRESSURE, OR HYPERTENSION?

High blood pressure is a pressure greater than 140/85. It is measured in millimeters of mercury (mm Hg). It is the most common cause of problems with the arteries – heart attacks, strokes, and heart failure.

WHY IS HIGH BLOOD PRESSURE DANGEROUS?

We need pressure in our arteries to push blood around the body If the blood pressure is too low, blood will not circulate. Imagine

---

the pressure in a garden hose used for watering the flowers. If the pressure is too high, for example, as high as a jet washer on full force, the water comes out as a jet and damages the flowers. If the water pressure is too low, it drips out of the hose and hardly wets the soil.

If our blood pressure is too high, the pressure inside the arteries puts a strain on the arteries, which become stiffer. The high pressure inside the arteries pushes globules of fat (cholesterol) into the walls of the arteries. The higher the pressure in the arteries, the harder the heart has to work to force blood around the arteries. If the heart has to work too hard for too long, the walls of the heart can initially get thicker, but after some time (usually a few years), the heart becomes weak and it fails. High blood pressure is the most common cause of heart failure. Once the heart fails, it cannot repair itself, although it can be controlled to some extent with medication.

ARE ALL THE ARTERIES AFFECTED BY HIGH PRESSURE?

Yes. High blood pressure affects mainly:

- the arteries supplying blood to the brain (cerebral), causing strokes.
- the eye (retinal) arteries, causing problems with eyesight.
- the heart (coronary) arteries, causing angina and heart attack.
- the aorta (the main artery coming out of the heart and from which all the other arteries branch off), causing blowouts or aneurysms, which can burst or rupture.
- the leg arteries, causing pain or discomfort in the calf of the leg or claudication when walking.

HOW IS BLOOD PRESSURE CONTROLLED?

The heart generates a pressure to push blood around the body. The pressure is mainly controlled by the width or diameter of the smaller, elastic arteries called arterioles. The wider they are, the lower the pressure; the smaller and more narrow they are, the higher the pressure. The diameter of the arterioles is controlled by chemicals produced by the kidney and also by nerves, which make them relax and widen, or contract and squeeze down very quickly. Arterioles can change their width very quickly, which is why blood pressure can change, and must be able to change, from second to second.

IS BLOOD PRESSURE THE SAME ALL THE TIME?

No. It increases when we exercise in order to push blood and oxygen to the leg and arm muscles, and also when we are stressed.

The pressure is low when we rest, or after a heavy, relaxing meal, or when we sleep. This explains why if we stand up quickly or get out of bed quickly, we may feel faint. This is because the blood pressure is low while we are in bed. While we're in bed, our leg arteries are expanded wide open (dilated), and a lot of the blood is in our legs and feet, and takes time to get to our head when we stand up. Blood falls to our legs when we stand for long periods. Unless the leg muscles squeeze the blood in the veins back up to the heart, there is less blood circulating around the body to the brain. This can lead to fainting, particularly in hot weather when the person is dehydrated. This is why guardsmen stand up and down on their toes. This action squeezes blood from the leg veins back to the heart. It is also important to drink plenty of water in hot climates or if sweating a lot during sports.

Blood pressure varies a lot in everyone, depending on the weather, where they are, what they are doing or have been doing, and what they are thinking about.

9

> *Treatment for high blood pressure should not be started until the doctor is sure that the patient has sustained high blood pressure and is not simply overweight or inactive and/or drinking too much alcohol.*

HOW DO PEOPLE KNOW IF THEIR BLOOD PRESSURE IS HIGH?

Blood pressure doesn't cause symptoms. People will know only by getting it measured by someone who knows how to do it properly and by using an accurate machine. Blood pressure has to be recorded when patients are relaxed. Several readings may need to be taken over several months if there is a question that a person's blood pressure is high (more than 140/85).

WHAT TESTS ARE DONE FOR PEOPLE WITH HIGH BLOOD PRESSURE?

The most important thing is to make sure that the blood pressure really is high all the time. This may mean having the blood pressure measured several times over several months. Sometimes a 24-hour blood pressure recording is done; this is helpful by excluding "white coat hypertension." Most people feel nervous when seeing a doctor or having their blood pressure recorded. The 24-hour recording, ideally done during normal daily activities (apart from swimming or bathing), records the blood pressure every half hour. This gives a full picture rather than a snapshot taken when the patient may be rushed and very nervous.

How Do 24-Hour Blood Pressure Recordings Help Distinguish "White Coat Syndrome" from Real, Sustained High Blood Pressure?

This test is useful in finding out if a person has high blood pressure requiring lifelong treatment or has normal blood pressure except when they visit the doctor. The latter is called "white coat syndrome"–high blood pressure when a person has blood pressure checked by a doctor or nurse. The 24-hour blood pressure recording is helpful in distinguishing between sustained (all the time) high blood pressure and blood pressure that is usually normal but increases a lot with stress or anxiety. Patients having the 24-hour recording wear a blood pressure cuff around their arm, which is connected by a tube to a blood pressure box attached to a belt around their waist.

Why Is It Better to Measure Blood Pressure When People Are Relaxed?

It's no good having blood pressure measured when patients are stressed or have just exercised or rushed about.

WHAT IS AN ACCEPTABLE BLOOD PRESSURE?

Less than 140/85. The upper figure (140) is the systolic pressure in the arteries (systole is the phase of the heart cycle when the heart is squeezing or contracting, pushing blood around the body).

The lower figure, the diastolic level, is the pressure in the arteries when the heart is relaxing between beats and refilling with blood (diastole is the phase of the heart cycle when the heart is relaxed and filling with fresh blood from the lungs).

ISN'T THE HIGHER FIGURE, THE SYSTOLIC, MORE IMPORTANT?

No. They are equally important. Elderly people are more likely to have a high systolic reading because their arteries are hard and less elastic. So when the blood is squirted out from the heart, the surge of blood hits a relatively hard, inelastic surface (a rigid and sometimes chalky artery wall), and the pressure at the time the heart contracts is high. There will be more of a splash if you hose against a wall than against a soft rubber sheet secured by rubber bands.

Younger people have elastic arteries, and so the force of blood coming out of the heart is cushioned by their soft, distensible, elastic arteries. Young people with high blood pressure usually have high diastolic rather than systolic blood pressure readings.

If either the systolic or diastolic figures are high, then that person has high blood pressure (hypertension).

DO SOME PEOPLE NEED A HIGHER OR LOWER PRESSURE THAN 140/85?

Yes. Diabetics should have a blood pressure lower than 130/80 because they are at higher risk of getting coronary heart disease and having angina and/or a heart attack as well as a stroke.

IS THERE ANY DANGER IF THE BLOOD PRESSURE IS TOO LOW?

Rarely. Blood pressure lower than 100/60 can make people feel lightheaded if they stand up quickly or lift their head up after bending over. As long as the brain, heart, kidneys, and all the other important parts of the body are getting enough blood, it doesn't really matter how low the blood pressure is. People would feel lightheaded if their blood pressure cannot increase enough to supply their brain with blood when it needed it.

Low blood pressure is not a bad thing: it is usually a good thing because people with low blood pressure live longer than people with high blood pressure.

It is very rare for people to need treatment for low blood pressure. If the blood pressure is very low, there may be a medical cause for it or the person may be taking medication (prescribed or not prescribed) that lowers it.

Is It Dangerous if People Feel Faint When They Stand?

No. Some people who take pills for high blood pressure feel faint from time to time, usually when they stand up quickly or get out of bed without sitting on the side for a few seconds. They may worry that their blood pressure is too low. This is usually not a problem and can usually be avoided if they simply don't rush and instead get up a bit more slowly.

SHOULD ELDERLY PEOPLE HAVE A HIGHER BLOOD PRESSURE TO GIVE THEIR BRAIN MORE BLOOD?

No. High blood pressure in the elderly is dangerous and increases their risk of strokes or heart attacks. It used to be thought that they should have a higher blood pressure, but this is no longer thought to be the case.

WHAT ARE THE CAUSES OF HIGH BLOOD PRESSURE?

In over 90% of cases, the cause is not known.
Some causes are treatable:

- being obese or overweight.
- drinking too much alcohol.
- not doing enough exercise.
- narrowing of the arteries to the kidneys.
- a tumor in the adrenal gland (a small gland producing chemicals—adrenaline and noradrenaline, and aldosterone and steroids—all of which increase blood pressure).
- narrowing of the main artery leading out of the heart (aorta) at the top of the chest.
- severe kidney disease, which is both a cause and a result of high blood pressure.

All these causes of high blood pressure are treatable. If they are treated, the blood pressure may resolve. That is why it is important for all these conditions to be investigated.

CAN BLOOD PRESSURE BE MEASURED AT HOME?

Yes. The new automatic, battery-operated machines sold at a drugstore or over the Internet are usually reliable and accurate. They are easy to use and give reliable readings. In general, arm recorders are more accurate than wrist recorders. It is useful for patients to check the accuracy of their device and their technique of recording their blood pressure by asking their doctor or nurse to measure their blood pressure simultaneously.

IS HYPERTENSION THE SAME AS BEING "HYPER"?

Some people get confused between the word "hypertensive" and anxious, uptight, or "hyper." Feeling stressed or anxious is not the same as being hypertensive, although stress and anxiety do increase blood pressure.

ARE THERE SIMPLE THINGS PEOPLE CAN DO TO LOWERING THEIR BLOOD PRESSURE?

Yes. Very often, blood pressure falls when people lose weight, cut down the amount of salt they eat, and do regular, daily, vigorous exercise. If patients with hypertension try the following for two to three months, it is possible that their blood pressure will fall to a normal level:

- Cut out all alcohol.
- Do not add salt to food.
- Achieve optimal weight (a flat tummy).
- Exercise hard to get a sweat for 30 minutes every day.
- Identify the cause of major stress factors and try to reduce them.
- Stop smoking.
- Eat a healthy diet with fresh fruit and vegetables and avoid junk food and ready-prepared meals, which contain a lot of salt.

Table 9.1: Drugs Used to Treat High Blood Pressure

Drug	How it works	What it is good for	Side effects
Calcium blocker	widens arteries	blacks	puffy feet, flushing, headache
ACE inhibitor drugs with "-pril" at the end	widens the arteries	blockages in the arteries; effective with diuretics	dry cough
Water tablet diuretic bendrofluazide	causes salt loss from the kidney	mild cases used with other tablets	impotence, low salt level, gout
Angiotensin II antagonists drugs with "-tan" at the end	same as ACE I	same as ACE I	rare
Beta blocker atenolol drugs with "-ol" at the end	slows the heart	angina, stress	depression, impotence, slow pulse, cold hands, asthma, may cause diabetes
Alpha blockers doxazocin	widens arteries	men with prostate problems	dizziness

WHAT DRUGS ARE USED TO TREAT HIGH BLOOD PRESSURE?

There are several families of drugs, and within each family are several members that have more or less the same effects.

CAN WOMEN HAVE SPECIAL PROBLEMS DUE TO HIGH BLOOD PRESSURE?

Some women have very high blood pressure during pregnancy. They get swelling of their hands and feet and pass protein in the urine, which is detected in the lab or doctor's office with a dip-stick test. High blood pressure during pregnancy is called *eclampsia* and is a dangerous condition that can damage both the mother and the baby. The mother is usually admitted to the hospital for bed rest, monitoring, and treatment.

There are less severe cases of high blood pressure when the pregnant woman does not need to be admitted to the hospital but is given drugs to lower the blood pressure. The blood pressure often falls to normal once the baby is delivered, but a proportion of women who have high blood pressure during pregnancy develop high blood pressure at a relatively young age later.

Women with high blood pressure in pregnancy are looked after by their internist, gynaecologist, and, often, a cardiologist, too.

CAN WOMEN WITH HIGH BLOOD PRESSURE HAVE A BABY?

Yes. They will need to see their doctor and gynaecologist to discuss the risks, but most women with high blood pressure can take a drug that is effective in controlling blood pressure and is not dangerous to the baby, thus allowing them to have a normal delivery. The key things are for them to be fit, not to smoke, to have a healthy diet, and to make sure that their blood pressure is monitored and well controlled on the correct drug(s).

IS THE ORAL CONTRACEPTIVE PILL DANGEROUS IN WOMEN WITH HIGH BLOOD PRESSURE?

Yes. The Pill can increase blood pressure, and so women with hypertension may need to change their Pill to a different type or may need to come off the Pill altogether and use a different form of contraception if the blood pressure remains high.

IS HRT SAFE IN WOMEN WITH HIGH BLOOD PRESSURE?

Yes. hormone replacement therapy does not increase blood pressure.

SMOKING

Read this chapter to learn that smoking:

- is dangerous and causes, besides lung and other cancers, heart attacks, angina, narrowing of the leg arteries, and strokes.
- is more common in people of a lower socioeconomic class and lower educational status.
- is becoming more common in girls and boys.
- can quickly become an addiction.
- is the single biggest cause of death, disability, preventable illness, and unnecessary health expenses in the United States and Great Britain.
- causes chronic bronchitis and emphysema.
- shortens the lifespan by 10 years.

IS SMOKING AS BAD AS IT SAYS ON THE PACK OF CIGARETTES?

It's worse! As well as increasing the risk of angina and heart attacks, strokes, narrowing of the leg arteries (claudication), lung cancer, bronchitis, emphysema, and other cancers, it takes away the sense of smell and taste, and it causes the skin to age prematurely and the hair to become hard and dull. Smoking makes the blood sticky and liable to clot in arteries. It discolors the skin and the nails, it smells, and to many people, it is unattractive. It is highly addictive.

Most smokers die of a problem related to smoking rather than another condition.

BUT ISN'T IT BETTER TO SMOKE BECAUSE IT REDUCES STRESS AND PREVENTS WEIGHT GAIN?

That's not true. Smoking is more dangerous than being stressed and worse than being overweight.

BUT WHAT ABOUT SMOKING ONLY ONCE OR TWICE A DAY?

Even that is dangerous. Two cigarettes are twice as bad as one, and even one a day is bad for the smoker and those near to him or her.

BUT WHAT ABOUT PEOPLE WHO SMOKED 40 A DAY AND LIVED TO BE 82 YEARS OLD?

Some people are lucky and can always cross a busy road with their eyes shut, and reach the other side, alive, in one piece. But most of us are not that lucky. Most smokers die younger than nonsmokers.

BUT IT'S COOL, RIGHT?

Not any more. And it's expensive.

SHOULD SMOKERS STOP SMOKING IF THEY'VE BEEN SMOKING FOR MANY YEARS?

Yes. After five years, their risk of disease is the same as someone who has never smoked. It's never too late to stop smoking. Although the best advice is not to smoke at all, the sooner smokers stop, the better and safer they will be.

> *Stopping smoking is the most beneficial thing that smokers can do to reduce their risk of death. People who continue to smoke are three times as likely to die than those who stop.*

People who stop smoking after a heart attack live longer than those who continue to smoke after their heart attack. Three years after quitting, the risk of having another heart attack is the same as in someone who has had a heart attack but who has never smoked.

People who continue to smoke after a heart attack double their risk of having another heart attack within a year.

Stopping smoking reduces the risk of problems of arteries narrowing after coronary artery bypass surgery and balloon angioplasty. Stopping smoking before heart surgery or any type of surgery shortens recovery time.

Most people who have claudication–pain in their legs when they walk–smoke or have smoked. It is essential for these people to stop smoking. If they don't, they run a big risk of losing a leg or both legs.

ARE THERE SPECIAL PROBLEMS IN WOMEN WHO SMOKE?

Smoking is more common among women than men. Smoking is just as dangerous in women as it is in men.

WHAT ARE THE DANGERS OF SMOKING DURING PREGNANCY?

Pregnant women who smoke are more likely to have a small, underweight baby born prematurely or have a stillbirth or lose their baby during pregnancy.

Babies born to mothers who smoke also have small body organs and their lungs don't work properly. They are twice as likely to die from a crib death. They are more frequently ill in childhood than babies born to nonsmoking mothers. They may become addicted to nicotine even before they start smoking, and they are more likely to become smokers, possibly because they see their mothers smoke. Children of mothers who smoke are more likely to be physically and mentally retarded.

Women who smoke and who are on the Pill are 13 times more likely to get angina or have a heart attack. Women should not take the Pill if they smoke.

10

IF PEOPLE STOP SMOKING, IS IT POSSIBLE THEY WON'T NEED A BYPASS OR ANGIOPLASTY?

Yes. Stopping smoking and changing your lifestyle (exercising, losing weight, eating a healthy diet) improve angina and may improve symptoms so much that smokers who quit may not need angioplasty or heart bypass operations.

PASSIVE SMOKING–WHAT IS IT AND IS IT DANGEROUS?

Passive smoking is being near other smokers and breathing in their smoke. Yes, it is dangerous. People who do not smoke but are in contact with other smokers or who live and work in smoky areas have an increased risk of getting coronary heart disease and cancer.

WILL THE LAWS ABOUT SMOKING IN PUBLIC PLACES MAKE MUCH DIFFERENCE?

Probably, but we will have to see how much of an impact they make.

DOES IT MATTER HOW MANY CIGARETTES A PERSON SMOKES?

Yes. The more someone smokes, the higher their risks of disease. Middle-aged men who smoke are two to three times more likely to have a heart attack and die compared to nonsmokers of the same age.

SO SMOKING REALLY IS BAD, BUT WHY?

The nicotine, the tar, and all the other dangerous chemicals in the tobacco and the carbon monoxide in the smoke, become even more dangerous when they burn and get hot. The tar causes cancer. Nicotine is also dangerous when cold. This is why chewing tobacco can cause all the problems of smoking cigarettes. Chewing tobacco is a powerful cause of mouth cancer.

The nicotine damages the lining of the arteries, making them thicker and narrower. Nicotine also makes the blood sticky and causes cracks in the layers of fat in an artery.

BUT SURELY, AREN'T LOW-TAR CIGARETTES SAFER?

Not really. Many people smoke more to get the same buzz. It's a bit like "low fat" food. These are words used by the companies whose profits depend on people buying what they believe to be a safe product! All tar is bad, and all cigarettes are dangerous, low tar or high tar.

ARE CIGARS BETTER OR WORSE THAN CIGARETTES?

It depends on how many are smoked and how big they are and what sort of tobacco is used. Cigars are as bad as cigarettes, and it used to be thought that one big cigar is as dangerous as 20 cigarettes.

WHAT ABOUT PIPES?

Pipe smoking is less common nowadays but may be more risky than cigarettes because smokers keep their pipe in their mouths so the tobacco, smoke, and all the nasty chemicals attack the lining of the mouth and tongue. This can cause cancer of the mouth as well as all the other tobacco-related problems.

HOW MIGHT SMOKERS FEEL IF THEY TRY TO QUIT?

After an initially difficult period, they will soon feel very much better. They will be liberated from their addiction, in control of their life, feeling more socially acceptable, and admired by friends, family, and colleagues. They will have more money to spend on other things (or save). Their sense of taste and smell will improve. This is why some people put on more weight; they enjoy their food more. This is often the reason why some people, particularly women, do not want to stop. There are ways to get around this, and their physician or nurse will often be able to help.

Some people do not immediately feel better, and feel depressed or down, irritable, anxious, bad-tempered, and restless, and may have difficulties sleeping.

These symptoms appear within a few hours, peak after a day or two, and last for several weeks – in some people for many months. Some people still have the urge to light up, years after stopping.

10

WHAT DO SMOKERS WHO HAVE TRIED TO STOP SMOKING SEVERAL TIMES, BUT COULD NOT SUCCEED, DO NEXT?

It all depends on how much they want to stop. If people want to do something badly enough, they will usually do it. The human spirit is amazingly strong. If smokers really want to stop, they will be able to.

But, as you know, it's not easy.

It is a lot easier if smokers who have been unsuccessful in quitting discuss this with the people they live and work with or socialize with. It is much more difficult and may be "impossible" to do it alone when other people around them continue to smoke.

The following 10 steps have been suggested and help some people quit:

1. Make a date and stick to it. Don't cut down, it doesn't work. Just stop completely.
2. Keep busy and throw away your cigarettes, lighters, and ashtrays.
3. Eat and drink sensibly and healthfully, and get plenty of sleep.
4. Tell your friends, family, and people you work with that you have stopped. Tell those who also smoke that you think it would be good for them to stop with you so that you can support each other.
5. Be aware of how you might feel when you stop smoking, and keep strong. Exercise every day. This is relaxing, and it destresses you and makes you feel generally and more emotionally strong and in control of your feelings.
6. If you used to smoke when you went to pubs or clubs or with certain people, stay away from these danger spots, however antisocial you feel. Remember, however awful it feels at the time, you will be more likely to give up if you remove yourself from the places where you used to smoke.
7. If someone offers you a cigarette, just say no. Smokers (like people who can't control their eating habits) are scared and envious about their friends or acquaintances who seriously try to stop. Seeing you work hard doing something useful, healthy, difficult, and brave makes them feel inferior and guilty.
8. Take one day at a time.
9. Remember, stopping smoking is more important than anything else you can do yourself to improve your health and reduce your risks of having a heart attack, a stroke, or lung cancer. Your health will improve from the day you stop.
10. Do it for yourself—you are the one person who has the most to gain.

> *If you succeed, you will feel great, in control, confident, and healthy, and you will be able to enjoy your life more. You will find it easier to concentrate and not have a sore throat and a cough. You will be able to breathe and move around more easily. You will live longer and enjoy the extra years you have gained by your hard work and mental strength.*

WHAT ABOUT SMOKING CESSATION CLINICS?

They work in 50% or so of people who attend them. Those most likely to be successful are those who really want to stop.

WHAT IS NICOTINE REPLACEMENT TREATMENT?

This is quite useful, but whatever form smokers take – spray, gum, lozenges, or skin patches—nicotine is nicotine! Again, the people who are most likely to be successful are those who are determined to stop. Some of these forms of nicotine replacement treatment are available by prescription. Some are available over the counter. They are not given to women who are pregnant or who breast-feed.

Smokers wanting to quit should choose the product they find most acceptable. These products are all equally effective.

The gum or spray is useful for people who have cravings.

Nicotine replacement treatments give a lower nicotine level than cigarettes and increase the chances of quitting.

Nicotine treatments are generally safe and, for patients who have had a heart attack, safer than cigarettes.

- *Patches*

  These look like sticking pads and are stuck on the arm or nonhairy skin. They last around 16 hours and come in three strengths, delivering nicotine slowly into the bloodstream through the skin. They are normally used for three months, starting with the highest dose patch and reducing the dose slowly. The patch can cause itching, so changing its position can help stop the itching.

  They are particularly useful for moderate smokers (10–20 cigarettes per day) and improve the chances of quitting by 50%.

- *Gum*

  This is useful for heavy smokers with cravings. It comes in different strengths. Many ex-smokers get addicted to the gum and find it enjoyable, but it is less dangerous than cigarettes. Do not chew more than 15 pieces per day. It should to be chewed and then left in the space between the gum and teeth for 30 minutes.

  It can be bought over-the-counter.

- *Nasal spray*
  It can be used 32 times per day. The spray gives a quickly absorbed "fix" and is designed for people with cravings.
  The spray can irritate the nose and throat.
- *Tablets and lozenges*
  These are similar to gum and are preferred by people whose teeth or dentures make gum difficult to use.

Bupropion (Zyban)

These tablets do not contain nicotine. They are aimed at people who want to stop smoking but are dependent on nicotine. They are best used as part of a smoking cessation program. This support service is an important part of the treatment. They work by reducing the desire to smoke and help reduce withdrawal symptoms. They double the chances of success in quitting.

Most people tolerate Buproprion, and it is quite effective. It is available by prescription, and the treatment is for 2 to 3 months. Side effects include a dry mouth and difficulty sleeping and headache, but these disappear after a few weeks. Buproprion is not given to patients with seizures, eating disorders, or kidney or liver problems or to women who are pregnant or breastfeeding.

ARE THERE COMPLEMENTARY TREATMENTS TO THOSE JUST LISTED?

Unfortunately, hypnosis, acupuncture, and special therapies (aversion therapy, making smokers scared of smoking) have not been shown to be effective. They are also expensive.

STRESS AND CORONARY HEART DISEASE

Read this chapter to discover that:

- stress affects everyone.
- stress is just as bad for your health and your heart as other cardiovascular risk factors.
- severe stress can trigger heart attacks.
- people who are stressed are often depressed.
- depression is bad for the heart, increasing the risk of coronary heart disease, and is bad for people who have had a heart attack.
- marital stress increases the risk of coronary heart disease.
- stress at work is bad for the heart.
- reducing stress with exercise, a healthy diet, and other methods is effective and improves prognosis in patients with coronary heart disease.

WHAT IS STRESS?

We all know when we are stressed and what it feels like. It is a feeling of being out of control and being under unpleasant, seemingly unending pressure. Many situations cause stress and may be related to illness, bereavement, work problems, career issues, family relationships, personal relationships, financial affairs, and most aspects of daily life.

Depression is usually part of stress and affects children, adolescents, as well as adults of all ages.

CAN STRESS BE MEASURED?

No. Unlike blood pressure, cholesterol, weight, blood sugar, or the number of cigarettes a person smokes, stress cannot be measured. Only the person affected knows how severe the stress is. It is subjective.

IS STRESS DANGEROUS?

Yes. Stress is dangerous for health and emotional well-being and bad for the heart. Certain forms of stress increase the chances of developing angina. Severe stress can trigger heart attacks.

HOW DO PEOPLE LEARN TO COPE WITH STRESS?

By experience and their own defense mechanisms. Coping with stress is difficult. We all get stressed at various times during our lives. We are not prepared for it when it hits us, and most of us have not been taught how to deal with it. Ideally, we should be taught to be prepared for it and how to cope with it when we are young. In the same way as children are taught how to swim to avoid drowning, they should also be taught what life situations may cause stress, how to recognize stress before it strikes, how to prevent it, and what to do when it begins to affect health and peace of mind.

> *One man's severe stress may be another's stimulation and challenge.*

IS IT STIMULATION OR STRESS?

When we are confronted by interesting and sometimes taxing and difficult challenges, which at first sight may be a little worrying or frightening, and we cope successfully by working hard and efficiently (if it is a task) or by controlling our emotions and behavior (if it was an interpersonal or emotional problem), that experience is rewarding and educational and makes us feel good; it reinforces our self-confidence. The challenge was stimulating and, ultimately, enjoyable. The stress turned out to be good. We coped. We came through it. We managed. We have learned something and are stronger for the experience.

But it may not always be like that, and we may not always cope.

WHAT DOES STRESS FEEL LIKE?

We all react differently to stress. One person may consider a situation, for example, an interview or exam, as trivial and nonstressful, whereas the same situation may be traumatic for someone else.

Therefore, how we react depends on whether we feel the stress is mild or severe and how long it lasts.

- **Mild stress**

  Mild stress for many people may be the frustration of being delayed in a traffic jam, a delayed flight, an exam, a job interview, or an oral presentation at work. The excitement of a first social date may transform to an unhappy relationship, which may be a cause of stress and depression. Personal and family relationships are a common cause of stress.

  Mild forms of stress may lead to a feeling of being on edge and not being able to completely relax because we have things on our mind. Fatigue and panic attacks are common. The common features of mild stress are generalized anxiety, loss of good humor and our sense of fun, and loss of interest in family, friends, and colleagues. The stress is a distraction, so the quality of our work may suffer. Some people lose their ability to relax and their interests in hobbies. Many people drink alcohol, smoke more cigarettes, take drugs, and either eat much more or lose their appetite, to counteract the effects of stress. None of these methods addresses the cause of the stress or help in the long term.

- **Severe stress**

  Major stressful situations affecting the core parts of our lives, and over which we have no control, affect the way our body functions. If stress is severe and lasts a long time, it makes us feel unwell, unsettled, uneasy, anxious, worried, angry, bitter and, in extreme cases, fearful and insecure. The stress affects our appetite, sleep, bowels, emotions, creativity, concentration, ability to enjoy life, sense of humor, reactions to other people, and sex life.

  Stress makes us feel unwell, weak, run down, fed up, and unable to join in the fun; even simple things like good food, sunny weather or an interesting TV program are not appreciated or enjoyed. Severe stress often makes us lose interest in our appearance and pride in how we look and present ourselves.

11

WHAT ARE THE SYMPTOMS OF THE STRESS SYNDROME?

The symptoms (pieces) that commonly make up the stress syndrome are the following:

- exhaustion, overall fatigue, lack of mental and physical energy
- loss of sexual interest and decreased libido
- irritability, being short-tempered
- anxiety, fear, dry mouth
- panic attacks – sweaty palms, heart pounding (palpitations), loose bowels, nausea
- sadness; loss of appetite, sense of humor, and fun; crying
- disinterest in family, friends, and colleagues
- forgetfulness, poor concentration, disinterest in hobbies
- difficulty sleeping, waking up early in the morning
- lack of ambition, purpose and direction: "everything is pointless, nothing matters, things couldn't be worse"
- lack of interest in life, no interest in fun things, hobbies, sports, current events, gossip
- muscle and joint aches, headaches, chest pain, breathlessness
- needing or wanting to be alone
- sweating
- bowel disturbances, with diarrhea
- nausea.

WHAT IS THE RELATIONSHIP BETWEEN DEPRESSION AND STRESS?

Depression affects nearly everyone, to different degrees, at some time in their life. People who are stressed are often depressed. Depression is a cause of both physical and social problems. Depression becomes more common as we get older. It is more common in women, Blacks, people who are not well educated, single people, smokers, and those who are physically inactive. The typical features of depression are having:

- feelings of being down, "can't be bothered"
- a decreased interest in all activities lasting for more than two weeks
- a change in appetite
- sleep disturbances
- fatigue

- agitation
- feelings of guilt or worthlessness
- difficulty in concentrating
- suicidal thoughts.

WHAT ARE THE EFFECTS OF DEPRESSION ON OUR BODY?

Our normal body functions become disturbed. This may lead to diarrhea and needing to pass urine more frequently, low sex drive and poor sexual performance, and loss of interest in our partner or spouse and family. We perform below our best at home and at work.

HOW CAN DEPRESSION BE RECOGNIZED?

There are two types of depression, major and minor.

Major depression
Having persistently low spirits or loss of interest in most activities for at least two weeks, including at least *five* of the following:

- loss of weight or increase in weight
- altered sleep patterns (waking up early in the morning or having difficulty getting back to sleep)
- lack of energy
- poor concentration
- agitation and nervousness
- feelings of worthlessness and low self-esteem
- suicidal ideas.

Minor depression
This is diagnosed with the presence of *three* or more of the above, lasting for more than two weeks.

11

IS THERE A RELATIONSHIP BETWEEN DEPRESSION AND CORONARY HEART DISEASE?

Yes. Depression is bad for the heart:

- Depressed people are twice as likely to get angina and have heart attacks.
- A large proportion of patients are depressed to some extent after a heart attack or after bypass surgery.

- People who have had a heart attack are more likely to have another heart attack if they are depressed.
- Severe depression is as serious as having a weakened heart after a heart attack. Even mild depression is bad.
- Depression increases the risk of death in people who have coronary heart disease.
- Depression increases the risk of problems after coronary artery bypass surgery.
- Depressed people are less likely to look after themselves and change their lifestyle.

HOW IS DEPRESSION TREATED?

Most depressed people are stressed. Recognizing the cause of the stress and the depression is half the battle. The next part is to get generally physically and emotionally fit so that depressed people are able to cope better and think their way out of the stress and depression. Although not everyone is completely successful and may need professional help and support, many people can do a lot to help themselves.

Cardiac rehabilitation courses are helpful in reducing depression in patients after heart attacks, possibly by helping patients cope with their stress better, reducing social isolation, helping them give up smoking, helping them with their diet, and providing emotional support. People who are depressed before a heart attack are likely to become more depressed after their heart attack and may neglect themselves. These are a high risk group.

There are several ways to treat depression. These include drugs, psychological therapy, and group therapy. It is very important that depressed people see their doctor for help and support. Depressed people may feel too unwell to want help. Their friends and families should do all they can to help them and ask them if they would like professional help.

Herbal remedies, for example, St John's Wort, are popular, but there is no clinical evidence that any of them work. Their effects may be due to a placebo effect (feeling better, despite rather than because, of the treatment). Some herbal remedies may also interact with heart medication and so are not recommended.

Effective treatment of depression improves quality of life.

CAN PEOPLE IN COMPLETE CONTROL OF THEIR LIFE FEEL STRESSED?

Probably not, but who is in complete control of their life?

WHO GETS STRESSED?

Everyone—children and adults of all ages, wherever they live and whatever they do. Nobody is spared from stress. Even the most apparently stress-free individual probably experiences stress at some time. Even people who are thought not to have a care in the world have stresses and strains, anxieties and pressures, even those who you think are in complete control of their lives.

- **Stress due to personal problems**

  It affects people of all backgrounds and "social class." One person's stress may be considered a trivial irritation to someone else. For example, the loss of income in a factory worker or shop assistant with a young family may cause terrible stress, family tension, and anxieties, whereas to another person, who has no financial worries and no dependents, might be seen as an opportunity for rest and a vacation.

  Stress is part of everyday life and being with other people. It is getting up on time in the morning, the hassles, discomfort and irritations of traveling to work, facing unforeseen and unwanted problems upon arriving at work, disagreements or feelings of things being unfair at work, and hard work not being recognized and adequately rewarded. It is an inevitable part of working with other people, whether this is in school, a store, a factory, any kind of office, the hospital, a restaurant, a religious institution, or anywhere else.

  Some people, for example, politicians, may choose their career because they wish to be surrounded and exposed to the culture, antics, and behavior of other like-minded people, whose career depends on showing political superiority over their colleagues (competitors).

  Ambitious people tend to work in competitive fields and therefore work with other ambitious people. Competing is stressful and the environment, by its nature, creates winners and losers. People may avoid stress or run away from it and change their careers to escape it. The high-flying city worker or senior lawyer may well envy the life of a farmer or the

11

independence of a plumber. For many, the "grass is always greener" until they experience the alternative. For many people, stress is an inescapable part of their lives no matter what they do. Being stressed may be part of a person's personality.

> **Stress is part of life and is "other people." We all get stressed.**

- **Stress because of loneliness**

Stress and depression are very common and a major health and social issue in lonely, socially isolated people, particularly the elderly (most of whom are widows), the bereaved or physically infirm, and increasingly commonly, those who are separated or divorced. For some, this is less stressful than their previous relationship.

Shy people who do not mix well with others may be more stressed and depressed than people who are energetic and socially active and gregarious.

Elderly people who have to contend with the loss of a spouse or companion and other friends may find this depressing, stressful, and an unwelcome reminder of their own vulnerability.

WHY DO SOME PEOPLE COPE BETTER THAN OTHERS?

We do not know why some people can soak up stress like a sponge and others are knocked down by it and become ill. It may have something to do with personality, sensitivities, physical and mental strength, intelligence, upbringing and education, support from friends and family, the way one has learned to cope with pressures while growing up, and how much one cares about certain things. Much of it may be part of a person's personality, but this is not well understood.

But if you think that a person who strolls around, seemingly without a care in the world, is free of stress, anxiety, and pressures, you are wrong! It's just that you don't know the person well enough to know what they feel inside. Their stress may be mild and manageable, but there must be something on their mind or something in their life that they would want to change.

STRESS FROM PEER PRESSURE – WHAT DO OUR FRIENDS AND COLLEAGUES THINK OF US?

- **Childhood and adolescence**

    Peer pressure is a common cause of stress, anxiety and, occasionally, depression throughout life. Most people, and certainly young people, care a lot about how their peers see them. Children are sensitive to what their peers call them and the way they are talked about. Many children feel stressed and depressed about peer pressure and bullying, and they consequently develop inferiority and self-doubt, which are common sources of stress.

    Young people often feel insecure about their physical appearance. This is thought to be more common in girls. Are we good-looking, slim, fit, cool, well-dressed, talented, sporty, clever, self-confident, and surrounded by lots of friends?

    Some young people are left badly battered and damaged after a stormy, self-conscious, anxious, and embarrassed adolescence. It is not known whether children who are bullied at school and have had significant stress are more likely to develop heart disease. Peer pressure is a major influence among children and adolescents wanting to be part of the gang and not be seen as a geek or "loser" by others.

- **Adults**

    Adults are not immune from peer pressure as a cause of stress. Adults have had more experience, most have more self-confidence, and they may have greater social support (friends, families, and escape mechanisms) than children. Nevertheless, career, social, family, relationship, and financial pressures are common causes of stress and unhappiness.

11

HOW DOES SOCIAL SUPPORT COMBAT STRESS?

Warm and supportive relationships are a very effective buffer against stress for people of all ages. A strong social network of good, supportive friends provides emotional scaffolding and boosts morale.

Poor personal, family, school, and workplace relationships are a potent source of stress and depression and are often extremely difficult to control. The listening skills, support, and advice of a good, trusted, wise, and sensible friend can be very helpful.

HOW DOES STRESS START?

- **The bombshell**

  Stress can explode out of the blue, as in the case of bereavement, a sudden severe illness, or an unexpected financial or personal problem.

- **Creeping stress**

  Continuous aggravation and irritation concerning personal, domestic, or working life, with lack of control over the causes, may be the seedlings that grow into significant stress. Very often, several parts of life go wrong at the same time; this may cause rapidly increasing stress.

A new job may produce problems with living arrangements, separation from family and friends, and financial disadvantages and stress. This may cause unhappiness within the family and further stress. This may lead to further work stress. So the initial prospect of an exciting new chapter in a career may rapidly evolve into an emotional nightmare.

DOES STRESS HAVE THE SAME EFFECTS ON MEN AND WOMEN?

Little is known about the comparative effects of similar stresses in men and women. Severe job stress increases the risk of coronary heart disease in men but was not observed in a large group of female nurses. Whether it affects women in other types of jobs is not known.

It is often said, without any good medical evidence, usually by women who have been through natural childbirth, that women are able to cope with pain better than men. It is not known whether women cope better with stress than men.

In women who have had a heart attack, marital stress, but not work stress, increases the risk of further heart problems threefold.

ARE WOMEN MORE SUSCEPTIBLE TO STRESS THAN MEN?

It depends on how they live their lives and many other factors that are not well understood. These include emotional and physical strength, their disposition (whether naturally happy or sad), their experiences at home while they were growing up, their personal support structures (family, friends, partners), their social and financial circumstances, their work commitments, how they would like to live their life, and how they like to be regarded by others.

WHAT ARE THE PRESSURES CONFRONTING WORKING WOMEN TODAY?

Women today are probably more vulnerable to stress, strain, and depression than their grandmothers. This is because they are more likely to work in traditional male-oriented, competitive environments. There are more women in senior roles in professions and in business than there were 50 years ago. In Great Britain, more than 50% of medical students are female compared to around 15%, 30 years ago.

There is a much greater proportion of female chief executives, senior lawyers, partners in accounting firms, judges, and successful entrepreneurs.

If both family life and work pressures are excessive, it can lead to stress and guilt, both of which are major causes of depression and fatigue. This sets up the vicious cycle of stress.

There are more "house husbands" or men working from home with a greater childcare and domestic role. Only women, however, can give birth, and those who wish to continue their careers have to juggle all the different professional, business, and family duties and responsibilities. This may result in significant pressures and stress because they are doing several jobs at the same time.

11

IS STRESS RELATED TO STATUS AT WORK?

Any job may be stressful. Deadlines, lack of support, and grinding boredom at work may lead to stress. For example, a factory worker may be put under pressure to complete a certain number of tasks on an assembly line. A middle-level manager, responsible for the factory workers' completion of the work, may be under even greater pressure and may be even more stressed. Middle level managers are under much more stress than senior managers because of this "lack of control" and pressure from above. All professionals now work under greater stress and regulation and are more stressed than their counterparts 50 years ago.

IS THERE A RELATIONSHIP BETWEEN JOB STRESS AND THE RISK OF CORONARY HEART DISEASE?

It has been found that, for both men and women, stress at work causing high demands (job strain) increases the risk of coronary heart disease. The effects of stress are greatest among the young, more junior workers at a low level who are less powerful and less able to make decisions and delegate work.

The most junior, lowest-level workers, and the most senior are those with the lowest pressure and the lowest stress. The middle managers, who have to manage and take responsibilities for the lower grades and be accountable to their superiors to perform, are subjected to the highest stress and strain.

Job insecurity also increases the risk of coronary heart disease and heart attacks by increasing stress levels.

WHAT ARE THE RISKS OF WORKING HARD WITHOUT RECOGNITION?

Working without recognition is called "effort reward imbalance" and increases the risk of getting angina and heart attacks. It is more likely to be dangerous in people with low social support, who are lonely and depressed, and who are in the lowest employment levels. A good manager (and it is really part of good manners and consideration for the people you work with) will always thank staff and be polite, and encourage all those who work in the organization or business, whatever their rank. Looking after and encouraging staff, and recognizing their contributions, improves staff morale and their productivity, as well as improving their health. These aspects and attitudes of modern working practices sadly seem to have slipped in recent years.

DOES STRESS RESULT FROM TODAY'S INSTANT COMMUNICATION SOCIETY DEMANDING IMMEDIATE ACTION?

Electronic communications have replaced the gentle and less rushed, the "let's wait for the letter to arrive before we make up our mind and act too quickly" philosophy and way of doing business. Today, there is much less time to think before having to respond. Our correspondents, customers, and clients want instantaneous service and answers. Most people do not like waiting. But the immediacy of modern communications and the expectations that things must be done quickly are major sources of stress.

WHAT ARE THE STRESSES OF MODERN TRAVEL?

Leisurely travel and sightseeing remain a pleasant pastime for many people. Having to get somewhere on time is usually a hassle and, for many people, a major source of stress and an unpleasant part of their working day. Traveling in cities and to airports and using public transport at certain times of the day in cities contribute to tiredness and decreases the quality of life. It is not uncommon for people to get stressed driving on highways. It is not known whether travel stress increases the risk of heart disease.

ARE THERE GEOGRAPHICAL VARIATIONS IN STRESS?

It is recognized that people from different countries react differently to stress. These generalizations may be inaccurate in individual cases, but there does appear to be a pattern in big populations.

The northern European character has been described as outwardly unemotional, private, and stoical. They are caricatured as willing to complain only about politically neutral, inoffensive topics like the weather. Being unable or reticent to release and share tensions, anxieties, and concerns may contribute to stress. The problem has been reported to be even worse in northern Scandinavians, who have to survive and accept cold, short, winter days where there may be no sunshine for several weeks, and where winter suicide rates and alcoholism are increased.

It is not clear whether the warm, sunny weather, blue skies, colorful food, and the accepted, heat-enforced siesta after lunch, enjoyed by people living around the Mediterranean, result in lower stress levels compared to those living in northern Europe, but it should! The "don't do today what you can do

11

tomorrow" philosophy should also lessen the effects of pressure and deadlines as causes of stress.

Not all people living around the Mediterranean may have such enviable lifestyles, but it has been known for many years that coronary heart disease is less common in southern Europe compared to northern Europe. There are several possible reasons for this, including lower stress levels and a better, less dangerous, lower saturated fat diet (olive oil rather than animal fat or vegetable oils).

WHAT ARE THE BENEFITS OF SUNSHINE ON STRESS?

Most people do not feel as well or as happy going to work and coming home in the dark, cold, wet days of winter. They look forward to summer and their summer vacation to recharge their batteries; the sun warms up the spirit and the fresh air blows away the stress, at least until they return home. This emphasizes the therapeutic benefits of the sun and sea that have been recognized and sought after for many years as effective treatments for a variety of disorders.

WHAT IS THE RELATIONSHIP BETWEEN STRESS AND ILLICIT DRUG USE?

People take drugs for lots of reasons. People who are stressed may want to escape from reality because they cannot cope, and they may indulge in a variety of drugs. All illicit drugs are dangerous to some extent, but some are very dangerous. Cocaine may cause heart attacks and angina because it causes the heart arteries to clamp down very suddenly.

Drugs injected into a vein or artery are very dangerous and may cause a severe, and often fatal, infection of the heart valves called infective endocarditis. The infection occurs because the skin, drugs, syringes, and needles are not clean. The drugs may contain impurities.

Several drugs, particularly those like heroin, cause depression. The more depressed addicts get, the more heroin they need to take. This may lead to an overdose. Heroin causes the brain's breathing center to stop working, which is a common cause of heroin deaths.

Drugs cause mental illnesses other than depression. People who are profoundly depressed and stressed may also develop a mental illness called psychosis. They may be too ill to recognize how ill they are and why they are ill. They may not have the mental and physical strength to cope on their own. It is therefore very important that their friends and family help them seek professional help quickly.

People who engage in the drug culture usually have an unhealthy lifestyle; they do not tend to exercise or have a healthy diet.

WHAT ARE THE EFFECTS OF STRESS ON LIFESTYLE?

People who are stressed often have an unhealthy lifestyle, which may increase their risk of coronary artery disease.

- Smoking is a strong, independent risk factor for heart disease, lung cancer, bronchitis, and emphysema.
- Alcohol is fattening, increases the cholesterol and triglyceride fat levels, and increases the blood pressure. It is poisonous to the heart muscle, leading to heart enlargement, weakening of the heart muscle, and heart failure. It also irritates the heart, causing an irregular rhythm called atrial fibrillation, which may develop after a binge.
- Eating disorders are common. Some people eat for "comfort" and eat high-fat and high-salt junk food for comfort and convenience, while others do not eat at all or drink alcohol and eat little food.
- Stress makes some people drop their good habits. They may stop going to the gym for a variety of reasons, and other components of their healthy schedule lapse. The lack of exercise may also contribute to depression and further stress.
- Stress interferes with sleep, causing a knock-on effect.

OUR 10 STEP METHOD TO REDUCE STRESS

Step 1.   Identify what makes you stressed or depressed, and try to change it.
Step 2.   Remember that if you want to feel better, a positive attitude will help you will feel better, but it will not happen overnight.

11

Step 3.   Get physically and emotionally fit.

Step 4.   Get into a daily routine of eating a healthy, varied diet with no additives and that is low in fat and salt. Drink as little alcohol as possible. Stop smoking completely. Drink caffeine in moderation.

Step 5.   Exercise every day.

Step 6.   Get plenty of rest and sleep.

Step 7.   Surround yourself with nice, humorous, supportive people whom you can talk to.

Step 8.   Find something interesting in your daily routine. If you can't, consider changing the routine. Find a hobby or a project, working either alone or with supportive people whom you feel comfortable with.

Step 9.   If you feel tearful, sad, unhappy, desperate, or suicidal, speak to your doctor.

Step 10.   Whatever you do, do not give up. If the program works, continue. If it does not work, keep going; it will work eventually.

Living a healthy life may mean having to make big and difficult changes, and stopping some of the things you enjoy; some of these (for example smoking and drinking alcohol) you may believe are helping you to cope with stress. The things that will work, making you feel better, and reducing your stress and your risk of developing coronary heart disease are:

- Stopping smoking completely. Reducing the amount you smoke helps a bit because smoking even one cigarette per day is harmful.
- Reducing the amount of alcohol you drink. Alcohol is a depressant substance. Stopping all alcohol for a few weeks may be difficult. But if you do, you will feel better, fitter, less depressed, fresher, and more alert during the day and more able to concentrate. You will lose a considerable amount of weight if you had been drinking over 10 units per week, and your cholesterol, blood sugar level, and blood pressure will fall. They may fall low enough to make treatment of high cholesterol and blood pressure unnecessary.

- Eat a low fat, low carbohydrate diet with plenty of fresh fruit and vegetables and chicken and fish. Avoid processed or packaged foods, canned foods (other than canned fish), snacks with additives and salt, takeout, and fast food.
- Exercising, ideally, every day and doing a form of exercise that you enjoy and that you will continue for the long term. Going to the gym is not everyone's idea of fun, but it is not meant to be if you do it properly. Many people join a gym, go once or twice, and then resent having to pay the membership because they don't enjoy it, and don't return. Gym work does not need to be enjoyable, and the best exercise is one where you exert yourself. The idea is to get hot, sweaty, and breathless for at least half an hour, every day. Exercise to this intensity is useful. Useful exercise should be uncomfortable. Sitting around the gym refreshment bar is not exercise and does not decrease cardiovascular risk, although the social interaction and relaxation may reduce stress.
- Getting good-quality sleep every night. Stress and depression often ruin a person's regular sleep pattern, causing early morning wakening. This leads to fatigue, irritability, and further stress. It leaves you feeling too tired to cope and think clearly. Exercise at the end of the day improves the ability to get off to sleep and may help you sleep throughout the night without waking up. Some people may need a short course of a sleeping pill, but this is not recommended unless other methods have failed.

DOES STRESS, ON ITS OWN, INCREASE THE RISK FOR HEART DISEASE?

Yes. Stress is thought to be an independent cardiovascular risk factor. This means that people who are stressed, even if they do not have any other risk factor, are more likely to develop heart disease than those people who are not stressed. It has taken many years for stress to be identified as an independent risk factor, because it is difficult to measure and the effects of stress acting alone were difficult to separate from the other well-established risk factors. Stressed people may have high blood pressure, may smoke, may eat fatty food and be inactive and overweight, and therefore have high cholesterol and high blood sugar, or come from a family affected by heart disease at a young age.

11

HOW MAY STRESS AFFECT THE HEART?

Under certain stressful situations, the brain sends impulses to the two small adrenal glands that lie on top of the kidneys. They produce two chemicals called adrenaline and noradrenaline, which affect the body in various ways. These chemicals are released into the bloodstream to help the body react to stressful and potentially dangerous situations. This is often called the "fight-and-flight response." The heart rate and blood pressure increase, the breathing gets faster and deeper, sugar is released into the blood from the liver providing energy and fuel for the muscles, and the person feels sweaty and nervous. These chemicals can be measured in the blood. The brain senses, feels, hears, or sees the danger and the adrenal glands produce the chemicals that enable the person to either fight or flee.

High levels of adrenaline and noradrenaline in the blood for long periods increase the blood pressure, and this increases fat deposits in arteries. Sudden increases in these chemicals are thought to inflame the artery wall, causing cracking of the surface layer of the fat. Blood clots form on the cracked fat layer, blocking off the artery, and cause a heart attack.

WHAT DRUGS ARE USED TO BLOCK THE EFFECTS OF STRESS CHEMICALS?

Beta blockers are drugs (those ending in " –ol", like atenolol) used to block the effects of these chemicals and are useful in patients with angina, heart attacks, and high blood pressure and in certain people with a weakened heart muscle (heart failure).

WHAT TYPES OF STRESS ARE DANGEROUS AND INCREASE THE RISK OF CORONARY HEART DISEASE?

There is strong and consistent evidence that:

- depression
- social isolation
- lack of good social support

are all *independent factors* that increase the risk of coronary heart disease as much as fivefold in men and women of all ages.

These factors also worsen the outlook for patients who have coronary heart disease. People who have angina or have had a heart attack, angioplasty, or heart bypass surgery do worse and are more likely to die earlier if they are lonely and depressed, compared to people who are happy and well-supported. This may partly explain why depressed, isolated, elderly widows and widowers often die soon after the death of their spouse.

The risk from these psychological and social factors is similar to other conventional risk factors. Therefore, being depressed, lonely, or socially isolated is as bad for you and your heart as smoking, having high blood pressure, high blood sugar, or high cholesterol, or being overweight and not exercising regularly.

WHAT ABOUT PANIC ATTACKS AND ANXIETY: CAN THEY DAMAGE THE HEART?

There is no convincing evidence that these increase the risk of cardiovascular disease.

HELPING OTHERS CAN HELP OURSELVES

We are all very busy with our own lives, but visiting, supporting, and cheering up elderly relatives, friends, and neighbors is something we all can do. It does not need to take a long time. Just popping in to see how they are and giving them a smile are simple, cheap, and nice, kind things to do. Little things like this can make lonely people happy, and feel as if someone cares about them and that they are not alone.

Although there have been no studies proving that social clubs, outings, home visits, and supportive social networks reduce the risk of heart attacks in depressed, lonely people, it is likely that these things would work and make them feel better.

Helping others is a positive and useful thing to do. It helps us realize that there are people worse off than ourselves. Voluntary and charitable acts, which do not need to be financial, are useful, positive ways to counteract the sources of stress in our lives.

HOW ARE LAUGHTER AND GOOD HUMOR USED AS A STRESS BUSTER?

It would be odd, and probably unnatural and abnormal, for people to be too happy, laughing and joking all the time. It

11

would also be rather irritating to people around them. But there is some evidence that happy, humorous people are less likely to get coronary heart disease than miserable, humorless people who may be also very stressed. People with a sunny, happy disposition may have a lower cardiovascular risk than discontented people; they are more fun to be with and their good humor may rub off on the people they are with. A smile can be infectious to other people. It is very difficult to prove that happiness, laughter, and fun protect people from heart disease, but it is highly unlikely that they are dangerous.

WHAT ABOUT THE "TYPE A" PERSONALITY?

It was thought for many years that aggressive, competitive, rushed, impatient, highly ambitious, driving, and workaholic-type people with few or no interests outside work (the Type "A" personality) were at greater risk from heart disease. This is no longer thought to be the case.

CAN MILD FORMS OF STRESS TRIGGER ANGINA ATTACKS?

Yes. Watching your children compete at a sport, your favorite team play football, a thriller on TV, or a good film at the cinema; experiencing anger and frustration at work, at home, in traffic, or in a line; or having a frustrating telephone conversation or argument are all well-known, common triggers of angina in people with coronary heart disease. The excitement and tension quicken the heart rate, increase the blood pressure, and, in some cases, cause the heart arteries to go into spasms and close down. The blood and oxygen supply to the heart decreases, causing chest tightness. It usually passes off quickly when the person cools down or walks away from the stress, or takes a spray of their GTN (glyceryl trinitrate is a spray medication to relieve attacks of angina). Only rarely, and if the stress is severe, would these attacks lead to a heart attack.

> *It is important for people with coronary heart disease who know that they may get angina with certain predictable causes of stress, to try to avoid these situations and to take their GTN spray beforehand, or as soon as possible with the onset of the attack.*

CAN LIFE EVENTS OR STRESSORS TRIGGER HEART ATTACKS?

Severe stress and a feeling of utter frustration and lack of control may lead to a heart attack. Acute life stressors, including bereavement and sudden severe illness, breakdown in a relationship, physical trauma, significant financial and career events, and the much less common but catastrophic events of natural disasters, wars, or terrorist attacks can trigger heart attacks.

These severe stressful situations are often unpredictable and difficult to avoid.

> *People with coronary heart disease should go to the nearest Emergency Room if they experience severe, long-lasting chest pain, sweating, and breathlessness that do not pass quickly.*

IS A "BAD MARRIAGE" BAD FOR WOMEN?

Yes. Marital stress has been shown to increase the risk of coronary heart disease threefold in women.

WHAT ABOUT ANGER IN YOUNG MEN AND HEART DISEASE?

Men aged 30 to 50 who become angry at certain situations in their life have been shown to develop heart disease and heart attacks at a younger age (younger than 55). Therefore, ways to reduce anger and stress in young men may prevent premature heart disease and heart attack. Certainly, angry young men are more likely to die early from heart problems than men who are calm. It is well known that severe anger and rage increase blood pressure and heart rate, and it is thought that this may trigger heart attacks. Generally speaking, a cool and calm personality is healthier than a highly charged emotion. Young children and young adults can be taught to control stress, and react to stress and provocative life events in a more measured and calm way.

IS EFFORT REWARD IMBALANCE A CARDIOVASCULAR RISK FACTOR?

Employees who are treated as "second-class employees" feel demotivated, angry, disenchanted, and emotionally disenfranchised from their organization. This leads to poor performance. Office politics are common and, for some, a major cause of stress, which may lead to serious heart disease. This may lead to depression and physical illness. The victims of workplace prejudice very often adopt the attitude of "if they treat me like this, then I will have no respect for them and will not be committed to the organization."

Appraisals at work are intended to be a useful, productive, positive, two-way exchange of views between colleagues or employers and employees. This should reduce stress and have very beneficial results in reducing heart disease. There is no doubt that "effort reward imbalance" is of considerable public health importance.

High job demands predict the likelihood of heart disease. Therefore, employees put under stress with deadlines and overburdened with work they realize is unrealistic and unreasonable, are likely to get stressed and depressed. This is more likely among younger workers who are less likely to have the emotional or psychological experience and resilience to cope with these pressures. It is not yet known whether social support at work can reduce job strain. It would appear that the best way to treat job strain and high demands is to reduce these potentially very dangerous problems with good management.

ARE DEPRESSION, LONELINESS, AND LACK OF SOCIAL SUPPORT CARDIOVASCULAR RISK FACTORS?

Depression, social isolation (loneliness), lack of emotional support from family and friends are independently associated with heart disease and the risk of heart attack and death. This is very difficult to treat, as these people are "invisible" and unlikely to seek help. They may resort to drugs, alcohol, and, in extreme cases, suicide.

There is less support for these isolated people in today's impersonal and fragmented communities.

These conditions are common in the elderly, especially after the death of their partner or spouse. There are few things more depressing than loneliness, to a person who is frail and medically unwell and who has major financial problems. The bereavement may trigger a heart attack in an elderly, vulnerable person.

CAN SOCIAL INTERACTIONS AND NEW CONTACTS HELP LONELINESS?

The comfort, help, support, and new social contacts in a communal home can be a positive experience for many lonely and elderly people. They are given the opportunity to be with other people and, if equipped socially, may find new friendships and companionship. This may provide, for some, a new lease of life.

Friendship clubs and religious groups and services are a very useful way for elderly, single people to meet. Prayer and religious fortification are very useful ways to strengthen the spirit. Words of comfort, support, and humor are very effective ways to reduce depression and stress.

WHAT ABOUT FITNESS CLASSES FOR THE ELDERLY?

Keeping not only the mind but the body fit is very important. Therefore, exercise classes and the ability to walk, do gardening, swim and make this a part of the daily program, can reduce depression and stress. It is important that these are supervised by experienced staff and that the participants are well enough to engage in these activities. Flexibility, stamina, and strength are important.

SHOULD STRESS MANAGEMENT BE TAUGHT IN CHILDHOOD?

Children should be taught as soon as they are able to understand, that during their life, they will face major hurdles that they will have to climb over. Some people find these hurdles very low and others very high. Nevertheless, everyone has to get over them and most of us are strong enough to conquer surprisingly major and at first sight, insurmountable hurdles. There are no formal classes to learn these life skills, and we all learn as we go along. Most children are taught life skills by their parents and close family members. When children get to their teenage years, they may feel that their parents have nothing more to teach them.

WHAT ARE SOME COMMON CAUSES OF STRESS AND POTENTIAL CAUSES OF DEPRESSION, AS RISK FACTORS FOR CORONARY HEART DISEASE?

Starting school, changing school, leaving school, taking tests, getting into places of higher education, applying and competing

---

for jobs, being made redundant or being dismissed from your job, and finding new things to do are part of life and major causes of stress and sometimes depression.

Failed or broken relationships are a very common cause of stress, disappointment, and pain in people of all ages. One of the most painful experiences is divorce and marital breakdown, particularly when children are involved. It is stressful for the children, too, and can trigger major psychological disorders in any party. Some people never get over it. This chronic stress is recognized as a cause of heart disease.

CAN FINANCIAL PRESSURES CAUSE STRESS?

Financial pressures are common and may be a particular source of worry, stress, depression, and potential heart problems in people who are about to retire or who have retired. This is because they may not have a pension or an insufficient pension to survive. The problem has become worse because life expectancy has increased over the last generation.

Most people who do not have major cardiovascular risk factors, apart from age, can expect to live well into their 80s or 90s. Young people, who adopt a healthy lifestyle, have a high chance of living into their 90s.

Children and young adults should be taught about financial matters and discipline, so that they can manage their affairs when adults. This may avoid problems and stress later in life.

WHAT ARE WAYS OF COPING WITH AN ANXIOUS PERSONALITY?

People who are worriers and who are generally anxious about nearly everything in their lives, find many situations stressful. They may also have underlying depression or a true psychiatric illness. This may be related to problems during childhood, which will also need to be dealt with. It is generally very difficult to change a person's personality, but their anxiety can often be managed simply and effectively without medication. Behavioral therapy and counseling may be effective.

This does require a considerable amount of time and expertise. It is also probably under-recognized because people who worry and who are anxious feel that this is a personal problem and not a medical condition that can be helped.

Medication is rarely prescribed unless the condition is very severe and interferes with a person's ability to conduct his daily affairs. The medication may be addictive or have bad side effects.

The type of drug used to treat depression must be selected by a doctor. Some older forms of antidepressant tablets (tricyclic antidepressants), which are now not commonly used, can, in some people with severe heart disease, result in heart rhythm abnormalities. Some treatments make people feel giddy when they stand up because they lower blood pressure. The new forms of antidepressants used are generally very safe, even in people with heart disease.

There are many forms of complementary medical treatments that some people find very helpful. These include acupuncture, meditation, reflexology, and other types of treatments. There is, however, very little objective scientific evidence that these treatments actually work. If an individual finds a form of complementary medicine that does not involve drug treatment helpful, then this should be encouraged.

Nevertheless, it is now recognized that all forms of complementary medicine should be properly validated and investigated by conventional medical means. It is no longer sufficient for complementary medical practitioners to deny the importance of scientific trials simply because "if it works for my patients, then it must be good."

WHAT ARE THE TRAITS OF ANXIETY?

The general features of people who are anxious are as follows:

- sweaty
- short of breath
- heart beating fast or forcefully in their chest
- chest pain
- irritability
- oversensitive to other people's comments that previously would have been ignored
- shaking of the hands
- avoiding interpersonal contact such as meeting people or going out for dinner, wanting to be alone.

WHAT ARE PANIC ATTACKS?

Panic attacks are very common and more common in young people in both men and women. People feel that they are extremely ill, feel their heart beating fast and forcefully in their chest, notice a change in their breathing pattern, and may breathe very fast and deep (hyperventilation). Sweating, having a headache or intense fear, not wanting to leave the house (agoraphobia), wanting to run away into the open air, not being able to tolerate being in a room (claustrophobia), are other features of panic attacks. Some people may hyperventilate and lose consciousness.

HOW CAN PEOPLE PREVENT STRESS?

There is considerable and growing evidence that leisure activities, sports—particularly daily vigorous cardiovascular exercise—and a good, healthy diet with plenty of sleep, maintain a person's physical and emotional fitness. When people become drained, emotionally tired, and physically fatigued, they may be susceptible to colds, other infections, and possibly a decrease in their resistance to infection. Many of us know that when we are "run down" we are more likely to get an infection. This is often a chest or a urinary tract infection. This can lower our resistance and make us tired, depressed, and more vulnerable to the pressures of everyday stresses and strains.

WHAT IS THE RELATIONSHIP BETWEEN DOMESTIC STRESSES AND WORK?

This can sometimes be very difficult, particularly when relationships are strained. This may be for many reasons. Partners and spouses do not always get along. There may be small family disagreements, which spill over to dissatisfaction at work. Pressures at work can have major influences on relationships at home between parents, partners, and their children.

When one strand of a person's life is under strain, this puts pressure on other parts. It is, therefore, very important that people remain healthy, in control, cool, calm, emotionally fit, and physically strong. This is a central linchpin to being able to "ride the storm" of family or work pressures. Without health, one is less able to survive what hopefully are only temporary pressures or life events. This demands a fairly focused and very self-conscious daily regime of healthy eating and getting plenty of exercise and sleep. This seeds a feeling of relaxation and well-being and the inner strength and resilience to cope with often unexpected bumps in life.

HOW CAN COUNSELING HELP?

Many people today listen and give very helpful support to people who are under stress and find it extremely difficult to cope on their own. However, professional counselors may not be affordable to everyone. It is thus very helpful that a close friend or family member is able to listen and help.

Many people find it embarrassing or a sign of weakness that they seek professional help or "cry on someone's shoulder." This is a mistake. Simply talking to someone about your problems can have major therapeutic benefits. It relieves stress. A problem shared is a problem halved. Very often, expressing fears, anxieties, and frustrations about any issue can help people understand the problem and help them solve their own problems. Talking to a good listener (and there are very few good listeners around and it is a great art) is a very helpful way for people to understand their own problems and put them into perspective.

Group therapy is another useful way to share problems among a group of people. People sit together and are able to tell each other how they feel and what their problems are. Very often, people feel much better expressing themselves and their fears, and unburdening their problems. Other people in the group may give practical advice, but simply listening to other people's problems may put a person's own problems into perspective. This can be very reassuring. Other people may have had similar problems and will be able to provide very practical advice on how to cope. Unburdening stress is helpful. It works.

HOW CAN PEOPLE UNBURDEN PRESSURES AT WORK

It is very important for people to be told as soon as they start a new job and even during a lifelong profession or career at any stage, that they have the ability and freedom to approach their employer or manager if things do not seem to be working well or they finds themselves under pressure. If there are political problems and the attitude of the organization is not to help but to put further pressure on, then people will need to seek professional and sometimes legal advice. Very rarely is it worth sacrificing your health, and the welfare of your family, for a job.

> *Vacations, leisure activities, and strong family and social bonds are the rudders that keep your ship sailing in a straight line despite the storms of life.*

It is often said that busy people seem to be able to cope with everything. This is certainly true to a major extent, but even very busy, capable, energetic, and competent people have their limits. Therefore, we all have to continually review our priorities in life and make sure that we do not take on too much. As we accumulate more responsibilities and duties, or want to do more for ourselves or other people, including our family, we may need to drop certain activities from our schedule in order to function properly and fulfill our other obligations. It is not possible to do everything all the time. People have to decide what they really want to do and what matters most to them. Things that cannot be fitted into the schedule must be stopped. This may not need to be forever but certainly while you reorganize your life and other activities. Decongesting your timetable will help keep you de-stressed and in control.

In a way, we could all do with advisors, counselors, or close friends to whom we can confide our fears and anxieties and explain the pressures we are under. They act as a sounding board and can help us help ourselves by solving our own problems.

WHAT ARE THE GENERAL PRINCIPLES IN PREVENTING AND COPING WITH STRESS?

Identify the cause of stress. If there is something you can do about this, do it. If there is something you can do about it but feel inhibited, embarrassed, and reluctant or scared to do it yourself, speak to a good friend or professional advisor and formulate and design a plan.

If there are marital problems and you cannot speak to your partner, speak to a good friend, your doctor, your religious advisor, or a marriage guidance counselor.

If there are problems or issues at work that you cannot deal with yourself, speak to a good friend or find an advisor in a senior position who will give you practical advice.

If you have financial problems, get expert help from your bank manager, accountant, or close friend. Increasing your borrowing because of debt only makes the problem worse.

If you are worried about your health, see your family doctor.

HOW CAN YOU KEEP EMOTIONALLY AND PHYSICALLY FIT AND STRONG ENOUGH TO COPE WITH STRESS?

Get plenty of sleep. Do daily, effective exercise. Eat a healthy, balanced, low fat, low salt diet. Eat healthy food at home rather than snack or eat convenience foods from supermarkets or fast food outlets. Take time for yourself for regular leisure activities every day. Pursue a hobby. This may be a physical form of exercise like gardening, an outdoor sport, cycling, sailing, rowing, basketball, hiking, baseball, or soccer. Team sports are particularly therapeutic but difficult to arrange throughout the year. Take an interest and pride in yourself. Look inwardly for your good points and find these reassuring and a source of self-confidence. Avoid alcohol. Do not smoke. Take a break from work. Reduce caffeine – tea, coffee, chocolate. Drink water if you are thirsty.

WHAT IS THE PSYCHOLOGICAL APPROACH TO DEALING WITH STRESS?

Be positive and think of a way forward. Speak to friends and family. Make sure you know what you want to do. Do not lose your sense of humor. Set a time every day for yourself for leisure, exercise, rest, and thought.

11

12

Heart Problems in Women

Read this chapter to learn that:

- 10% of women aged between 45–64 years old and 30% of women aged over 65 years old have heart disease.
- In people between the ages of 45–54 years old, heart attacks occur in 6 times as many men than women.
- After the menopause, coronary heart disease is as common in women as in men.
- When women get angina, they are 10 years older than men, and 20 years older when they get a heart attack.
- Heart attacks are very unusual in young women less than 40 years old.
- One in three women dies from a heart attack.
- Two thirds of women never fully recover from a heart attack.
- Women who have had a heart attack are more likely to die in the first two weeks than men. Around 40% of women die in the first year after a heart attack, but this depends on a number of factors including age, the presence of risk factors, and the state of the heart arteries and the heart muscle.
- One in three women over 65 years old has coronary heart disease.
- Women are twice as likely to die from a heart attack or stroke than from any form of cancer.
- Coronary heart disease kills more women than men.
- Some risk factors, for example, smoking, diabetes, high blood pressure, and abnormal blood fats, are more dangerous in women than in men.
- Whereas men tend to have typical symptoms of angina (chest tightness and shortness of breath), symptoms in women are more often "atypical" (back pain, indigestion-like symptoms, discomfort in the tummy). This makes heart problems more difficult to diagnose in women.
- Women tend to dismiss these symptoms, so by the time they see their doctor the condition is often more advanced and therefore more difficult to treat.

- Hormone replacement treatment (HRT) does not protect women against coronary heart disease.

SHOULD WOMEN BE CONCERNED ABOUT CORONARY HEART DISEASE?

Yes.

There are two commonly held myths:

1. Many people think that coronary heart disease is a male disease. This is not true. Although coronary heart disease affects women around 10 years later than men, in people over 65 years old, it is as common in women as in men. It is not understood why it occurs later in women.
2. Most women believe that they are more likely to die from cancer (breast cancer is the most common). This is not true. Women are four times as likely to die from a heart attack than from breast cancer.

> *Coronary heart disease affects women as much as men in people over 60 years old.*

WHY DOES CORONARY HEART DISEASE OCCUR LATER IN WOMEN AND DEVELOP SO RAPIDLY AFTER THE MENOPAUSE?

Coronary heart disease symptoms usually start around 10 years after the menopause, but the process of clogging of the arteries (atheroma) starts much earlier. It is thought to start in some people during childhood, particularly in those with an unhealthy lifestyle.

It has been suggested that women are protected by the hormone estrogen while they still have periods. After the menopause, when women go through their "change," the estrogen levels fall, and women become vulnerable to coronary heart disease.

After the menopause, coronary heart disease can progress very rapidly, particularly in women with cardiovascular risk factors. After the menopause, the levels of cholesterol, the "bad" LDL cholesterol, triglycerides, glucose, and blood clotting factors (fibrinogen) increase. All the substances increase the fat deposits in arteries. The way the blood vessels contract and relax also becomes abnormal.

SO WHAT SHOULD GIRLS AND YOUNG WOMEN DO TO REDUCE THEIR RISK OF HEART DISEASE?

Young women should do everything they can to reduce their risk of getting coronary heart disease and make sure that they stop or do not start smoking; that their blood pressure is normal; that they do not have diabetes or high cholesterol; that they are slim and fit. They should adopt good habits when they are young. After the menopause, women should be especially careful and have a healthy lifestyle.

> *Prevention of coronary heart disease should start in childhood, and young women should be aware of the risks they face if prevention is left too late.*

> *All women, particularly those who have had a heart attack and who are at increased risk of another problem, should be see their doctor and have all their risk factors checked. They may need medication and will need to be careful about their diet and their weight, and take advice about regular exercise.*

ARE RISK FACTORS MORE POTENT IN WOMEN THAN MEN?

Yes. Nearly all the risk factors such as smoking, high blood pressure, abnormal blood fats, and diabetes are, individually, more potent in women than in men. So, for example, smoking is more dangerous for a woman than for a man. Women with diabetes are more likely to die from a heart attack than a man of the same age who has diabetes.

Women with more than one risk factor are at even greater risk than men with the same risk factors.

12

> *The same risk factors apply to men and women but are more dangerous to women.*

IS CORONARY HEART DISEASE BECOMING MORE COMMON IN WOMEN?

Yes. This is probably due to changes in the way they live their lives. Generally, nowadays, compared to their mothers and grandmothers, women:

- smoke more than they used to
- work in stressful jobs and for longer periods of time
- are key contributors to family finances and may be the main source of income
- are more stressed
- have a diet that is higher in fat and salt
- drink more alcohol
- do less exercise and are more overweight
- are more likely to be obese and have diabetes
- continue to have their domestic duties and responsibilities and therefore have more pressures to deal with.

HAVE THE CHANGING ROLE AND INCREASING RESPONSIBILITIES OF WOMEN LED TO INCREASED STRESS?

A greater proportion of women are working in traditional male occupations, managerial posts, and professions, compared to women in their grandparents' days. These changes have come about due to several changes in society, including a realization that women are able to make major contributions in all walks of life. Pressures from women for equality in the workplace as well as families' needs to have two incomes are also factors.

HOW DO INCREASED STRESS AND TIME PRESSURES LEAD TO LESS EXERCISE, AN UNHEALTHY DIET, AND OBESITY?

Women have not lost their unique ability to have children, and there is a biological time window for this, usually coinciding with an important phase in their career. Most women still have the additional, busy yet traditional job of being the chief homemaker. Therefore, they have to juggle their commitments and responsibilities, which often leads to stress, fatigue, less time to look after themselves, less time to "de-stress," and less opportunity to exercise.

An unhealthy high fat, high salt, quick, convenience food diet leads to obesity and associated diabetes and high blood pressure. These important risk factors are more potent and dangerous in women and, particularly after the menopause, may lead to coronary heart disease. Coronary heart disease is increasing in women more than in men. Therefore, it is possible that in the future, coronary heart disease may become more common in women than in men.

> - *Angina and heart attacks may become more common in women than in men because risk factors are more risky to women, and women become more vulnerable after the menopause.*
> - *Women can reduce their risk of coronary heart disease by doing everything they can, starting from a young age, to reduce their risk factors.*
> - *The only person who can make these changes is the woman herself.*

IS STRESS MORE DANGEROUS TO WOMEN THAN MEN?

Although the well-established risk factors appear to be more dangerous to women than to men, it is not clear whether stress and work pressures, are also more powerful risk factors in women. If so, this would not necessarily mean that women are weak and can't withstand the pressure. Stress may also be one of the risk factors, along with diabetes, high cholesterol, and smoking, that pose a greater danger to women than men. The reasons for these risk factors being more dangerous to women are not known. Work and domestic pressures in both men and women are complex and difficult to measure and distinguish from other risk factors (see Chapter 11).

12

IS CORONARY HEART DISEASE MORE LIKELY TO BE DIAGNOSED IN WOMEN TODAY THAN BEFORE?

Yes. But it is not clear whether this is due to the heightened awareness among doctors and women that coronary heart disease is as much a female as a male condition. Doctors and nurses are now doing a lot more screening for cardiovascular risk factors and offering advice, support, and treatment to patients with abnormal results. This strategy appears to be working, and heart attacks are becoming less common.

WHAT ABOUT WOMEN AND SMOKING?

Smoking increases the risk of blockage in the leg arteries (peripheral vascular disease) sevenfold and increases the potential of coronary artery disease and myocardial infarction fivefold (Chapter 10). Even passive smoking is dangerous. Although the proportion of male and female adult smokers has decreased over the last three decades, smoking has increased among girls. Twenty-five percent of women smoke, and many of these are very young, damaging their heart and lungs, sometimes irreversibly, at an early age.

Many women get angina and heart attacks for no other reason than smoking. Women who smoked more than 15 cigarettes per day and used "high-dose" estrogen oral contraceptives (now rarely prescribed) were found to have a 20-fold increase in coronary heart disease risk. Passive smoking increases coronary risk in men and women by 30%.

HOW COMMON IS HIGH BLOOD PRESSURE (HYPERTENSION) IN WOMEN?

High blood pressure is unusual in young women and usually occurs together with other cardiovascular risk factors, for example, obesity, diabetes, and a high cholesterol level. High blood pressure increases the risk of heart attacks and strokes (Chapter 9).

High blood pressure is more common in women after the menopause possibly because they are older.

Women with high blood pressure are at least three times more likely to develop coronary heart disease than women with normal blood pressure. High blood pressure is more dangerous in women than in men.

WHAT ABOUT WOMEN AND DIABETES?

Diabetes is a common condition where there is too much sugar (glucose) in the blood (Chapter 8). Most adults do not know if they are diabetic. There are no symptoms of diabetes unless the sugar is very high and the patient is very ill. Like high blood pressure and high cholesterol, diabetes is a silent condition. Women who gave birth to a baby weighing over 10 pounds are more likely to develop diabetes later in life than women who gave birth to average-sized babies.

WHAT IS THE RELATIONSHIP BETWEEN WOMEN AND OBESITY?

This is a big and growing problem in many parts of the world. Being overweight increases substantially the risk of coronary heart disease and also increases the risk of strokes and cancer.

Children are fatter and less active than their grandparents. Many fat young girls (and boys) become fat adults. Just being overweight is bad enough, but people who are overweight often have high blood pressure and a high level of blood fats and are less likely to do regular exercise. All of these individual risk factors are even more dangerous when they exist together.

The more overweight a woman is, the more likely she is to have a heart attack. The type of obesity may also make a difference. It has been suggested that women who are fat around the tummy ("apple" shape) are more likely to suffer heart attacks then women who have relatively slim tummies but who are fat around the hips ("pear" shape).

Most women are concerned about their appearance and understand that being overweight is unhealthy. After the menopause, women become more vulnerable to coronary heart disease. They may feel less concerned about their weight and appearance. This is the time of their lives, however, when it is most important to be slim, active, fit, and supple.

12

WHAT HAPPENS TO PHYSICALLY INACTIVE WOMEN?

Physical inactivity is a risk factor and is a fundamental part of a person's lifestyle. People who look after themselves and exercise every day (or nearly every day) are usually slim, eat a healthy diet, have low cholesterol, and are rarely diabetic. On the other hand, people who do not look after themselves and who do not exercise, often have a variety of risk factors and are at high risk from coronary heart disease (Chapter 7).

Regular physical activity – at least half an hour every day to a level where we sweat and get breathless – reduces the risk of heart attack by at least 50%. The benefits of exercise depend on its frequency, intensity, and duration. The benefits of exercise apply equally to men and women, but the benefits may be greater in post-menopausal women, who are at greater cardio-vascular risk, than in pre-menopausal women. Therefore, young women should start exercising regularly and continue to exercise throughout their lives.

WHAT ARE INFLAMMATORY MARKERS IN THE BLOOD?

There is a protein in the blood called "C reactive protein." High levels are found in the blood in people with infection or inflammation. The levels of C reactive protein increase with age and are higher in smokers. High levels may predict a future heart attack or episodes of angina. Levels are high in patients who have had attacks of angina. It is probable that the high levels reflect the general inflammatory process that occurs inside the heart arteries. Levels are also high in women after the menopause, but it is not known why. At this moment, we do not check this in the blood as a screening test.

WHAT SYMPTOMS SHOULD WOMEN BE CONCERNED ABOUT?

Symptoms suggesting angina:

- Chest tightness or discomfort, or an ache or heaviness in the chest, arms or back, or breathlessness occurring with exertion, housework, walking up hills or stairs, or with stress or emotion.
- Symptoms worse in cold weather, or after a heavy meal, or with stress or anger.
- Symptoms that start with exertion, last a few minutes, and gradually pass within 10 minutes of stopping exercise.

If in doubt, see your doctor.

Symptoms suggesting a heart attack:

- Heart attack symptoms are similar but more severe than angina, last longer, and are not relieved quickly by GTN (glyceryl trinitrate), an anti-anginal, under-the-tongue spray.
- Sweating
- Shortness of breath
- Sickness
- Feeling faint.

> *If you are worried about how you feel, dial for an emergency ambulance and go to the hospital. The doctors and nurses will be able to tell you if you have had a heart attack and you can be reassured; if there is nothing to worry about, you can go home.*
>
> *The sooner people with a heart attack get to the hospital, the quicker treatment can be given and the greater their chance of surviving and living a longer life.*

WHAT SYMPTOMS SHOULD WOMEN NOT WORRY ABOUT?

- pinpricking or stabbing pain in a small area under the left or right breast
- tender ribs
- long-lasting ache (more than one hour) occurring only at rest or relieved by moving around
- pins and needles in the fingers when waking up
- acidity and belching after eating.

WHY IS CORONARY HEART DISEASE MORE DIFFICULT TO DIAGNOSE IN WOMEN, AND WHY IS DIAGNOSIS DELAYED?

Doctors make a diagnosis of angina from the patient's description of her symptoms. Nearly everyone with angina has coronary heart disease. Very rarely, patients with other conditions may have angina but have normal heart arteries. Whereas men with coronary heart disease are more likely to have the typical angina symptoms of chest pain and breathlessness when they exercise, symptoms of angina in women are more often "atypical" and include back pain, burning in the chest, nausea, and fatigue: symptoms that would not usually prompt doctors to consider a heart problem.

12

In women, symptoms of both angina and a heart attack are more likely to be atypical and less obvious. Therefore, there may be a delay in diagnosis. Women with chest pain are less likely to be referred to a heart specialist and less likely to have further tests. If women's angina or heart attacks are not diagnosed, then patients will not have the right treatment.

> *Unless angina and heart attacks are suspected, the diagnosis and treatment will be delayed.*

ARE HEART TESTS DIFFICULT TO INTERPRET IN WOMEN?

Yes.

False positive tests are more common in women.

The most commonly performed initial test in assessing a patient for coronary heart disease is a stress or *exercise ECG* (Chapter 14). But the test is not perfect. For reasons that are not clear, this test may be abnormal in both men and women who have normal heart arteries. Around 20% of women and 10% of men who have normal heart arteries may have changes in their ECG, suggesting an abnormality during an exercise test. This abnormal (or positive) test result occurring in a person with a normal heart is called a "false positive." Women are more likely to have a "false positive" test than men.

Stress echocardiography is a newer test, which may be helpful in women who cannot exercise or if they have an ECG abnormality that complicates interpretation. A stress echocardiogram is performed by injecting a special drug into a vein in the back of the hand while doing an ultrasound (echocardiogram) of the heart. The drug has the same effects as exercise by increasing the patient's heart rate and blood pressure. The squeezing movements (contractions) of the heart can be seen on a TV monitor. If a part of the heart is not contracting normally, this could be because there is be a reduced blood supply to that part of the heart.

HOW IS A CORONARY ANGIOGRAM (INVASIVE X-RAY OF THE HEART ARTERIES) PERFORMED?

Injecting contrast into the heart arteries (coronary angiography) via a tube (catheter) placed under local anesthetic into the artery in the groin is the most accurate way to see if the heart arteries are blocked. Because it is invasive (the tube goes into the body and into the heart and the arteries), there is a small complication risk (1 in 1000 risk of heart attack or stroke). Occasional problems with the artery and a little bruising are quite common. Complications of angiography are generally no more frequent in women than in men.

The test is done in several situations and provides very helpful information that helps doctors decide on the best treatment for each patient.

IF ESTROGENS "PROTECT" WOMEN FROM CORONARY HEART DISEASE BEFORE THE MENOPAUSE, DOES HORMONE REPLACEMENT TREATMENT (HRT) PROVIDE PROTECTION AFTER THE MENOPAUSE?

Unfortunately, no. In women with cardiovascular risk factors, it may increase the risk of coronary heart disease. In the cases of women who are at a high risk, HRT may slightly increase the likelihood of heart attacks, strokes, clots in the lungs (pulmonary emboli), and breast cancer. It has been estimated that two of each of these problems result from treating 1000 women for one year with HRT. One serious event occurs per 100 women treated for five years.

SO WHAT IS HRT GOOD FOR?

It is recommended for women with bad menopausal symptoms, including flushing. It may slightly reduce the risk of thin bones (osteoporosis). Generally, in women who do not have symptoms, HRT does not make women less depressed, sleep better, be more sexually satisfied, interested, or active, or help their brain work better. There are always examples of women who are very pleased with their HRT and feel that it improves their hair and their skin. It is sensible for women to consult their doctor about these matters.

HRT should be started at a low dose and increased gradually until symptoms resolve. Patients should see their doctor regularly, with the goal of reducing the dose of HRT every six months to see whether it needs to be continued. HRT is not recommended for women who do not have menopausal symptoms.

12

WHAT ABOUT THE BIRTH CONTROL PILL? IS IT SAFE IN WOMEN WITH CARDIOVASCULAR RISK FACTORS?

Yes, the Pill is safe in women who do not have any risk factors and so is almost always safe in young women. But in women who have risk factors, for example, women who smoke, are fat, have high cholesterol, are diabetic, or have high blood pressure, the Pill may not be safe because it adds to the risk of heart attacks. A woman with more than one risk factor should probably not take the Pill and may need another form of contraception.

Birth control pills containing both an estrogen and a progestogen (the "combined Pill") are the most commonly used. Their advantages over a single–ingredient pill are that:

- they are reliable and safe
- they cause less bleeding, less pre-menstrual tension, and less breast disease
- there is a reduced risk of cancer.

The Pill can increase the risk of heart attacks and strokes in women:

- who have any cardiovascular risk factor, particularly smokers
- who are over 35 years old
- who are obese
- who have a family history (first-degree relative) of arterial disease.

Therefore, a woman who smokes is at greater risk from developing coronary heart disease than a nonsmoker. A woman with several risk factors is at much greater risk, and the risks of the Pill may be too high. The greater the number of risk factors, the greater the risk of cardiovascular problems.

> *The Pill should not be prescribed to women over 35 years old if they have one or more cardiovascular risk factors.*
>
> *Before starting the Pill, make sure that you have been checked by your doctor or the family planning clinic for all cardiovascular risk factors.*
>
> *Women who smoke or have high blood pressure, should either not take the Pill or should stop smoking.*

WHAT ABOUT THE PILL AND CLOTS IN THE LEGS (DVTS)?

The Pill increases the risk of blood clots in the legs (deep vein thrombosis, or DVT), particularly in the first year of use. This risk is much higher in older women (older than 35) and higher in women who are obese, because the risk of DVTs is higher in obese women.

> *Women should not take the Pill if they have had a DVT.*

HOW OFTEN WOULD A HEALTHY WOMAN, WHO IS NOT ON THE PILL, GET A DVT?

Rarely. Five in 100,000 healthy, nonpregnant, slim women who are NOT on the Pill get a DVT per year.

SO, WHAT IS THE RISK OF GETTING A DVT WHILE ON THE PILL?

The risk of DVT in women taking the Pill is 15 per 100,000.

ARE WOMEN DIFFERENT FROM MEN WHEN IT COMES TO TREATING CORONARY HEART DISEASE?

In some respects, yes. Although women with angina and heart attacks are treated in the same way as men, the results of treatment differ between men and women. Calcium blockers (tablets ending with–pine, e.g., nifedipine, amlodipine) may cause unacceptable ankle swelling in women.

IF WOMEN HAVE A RISK FACTOR, SHOULD THEY TAKE ASPIRIN?

No. Only if they have blockage in an artery or are diabetic.

12

All women who have coronary heart disease (or have had a stroke or have narrowing in a leg artery) should take 75–81 mg of aspirin a day unless they cannot tolerate it (tummy ache, previous tummy bleed while on aspirin, or allergy). Some doctors may advise people with high blood pressure to take an aspirin to reduce the risk of stroke but most don't.

If in doubt, consult your doctor.

WHAT ABOUT ANGIOPLASTY AND SURGERY?

It used to be thought that women did not recover as well as men after angioplasty or coronary artery surgery, but this is no longer thought to be true. Women *may* recover slower than men after angioplasty and coronary heart surgery, and this may be because they are unfit. In some cases, the results of angioplasty and coronary artery surgery are not as good as in men because women's heart arteries are smaller and technically more difficult to treat. Some women (and men) are left with an unsightly scar down the front of their chest and their leg (where the vein used for the bypass is taken) after a heart operation.

Generally, however, women do as well as men when it comes to angioplasty or coronary artery surgery when being treated for angina or heart attacks.

SO, WHAT CAN AND SHOULD WOMEN DO TO REDUCE THEIR CHANCES OF GETTING A HEART PROBLEM?

1. Understand that they are as likely as men to get it and that their risk increases after the menopause. Women should therefore take at least as much interest in their hearts and arteries as their breasts and wombs! All women should be as concerned about their cardiovascular health as men, and probably more so.
2. Stop smoking, whatever age they are. Help girls and women of all ages to stop smoking, and discourage girls from starting.
3. Get their cholesterol checked if they are post-menopausal or if they have a family history or another risk factor. The target total cholesterol is 5 mmol/l and the LDL cholesterol (the "bad" cholesterol that causes the problem in the arteries) should be less than 3.0 mmol/l. The LDL cholesterol should be less than 2.0 mmol/l, and the total cholesterol to HDL cholesterol ratio should be >6.0, in patients with arterial disease, high blood pressure, and diabetes.
4. Eat a healthy, low fat, low salt, diet with lots of salad, fruit, fresh vegetables, fish and lean chicken.
5. Be slim and fit. Exercise vigorously for 30 minutes per day to get sweaty and breathless. For women who can't, any exercise is better than none. Be as physically active as you can. Older or unfit women who are able to walk should walk quickly.

6. Get their blood pressure checked. If it is high, get down to their best weight and exercise; if it remains high, see the doctor in case they need tests and medication.
7. Get their blood sugar checked. If it is high, indicating diabetes, lose weight, avoid sugars and carbohydrates (pasta, rice, bread, chocolate and sweets, chips, and most high-calorie snacks), do daily exercise, and have the blood sugar rechecked. If it remains high, diabetes is possible, and this may need further tests.
8. If they feel uncomfortably stressed, try to identify the main cause of their stress and try to solve the problem. If this is difficult to do alone, think about getting advice from friends, family members, and people at work to reduce the stress levels to an acceptably low level. Stress is part of life and almost impossible to get rid of completely. If there seems to be no solution, and it seems that the stress will last for a long time, try to make the best of a bad job and try to find ways of coping with it in the short to medium term. Being healthy and fit, having a good diet, and sleeping well are all effective in helping people live more easily with stress.
9. Avoid illegal drugs and reduce alcohol (no more than 1 unit on any day).

WHAT ABOUT WOMEN WHO HAVE CORONARY HEART DISEASE—HAVE HAD A HEART ATTACK, ANGIOPLASTY, OR CORONARY ARTERY SURGERY?

They have to try even harder to reduce their risk of further problems. They should do all nine things listed above, but their total cholesterol should be less than 4.0 mmol/l and their LDL less than 2.0 mmol/l.

12

Impotence and Sexual Aspects of Coronary Heart Disease

Read this chapter to learn that:

- Impotence (erectile dysfunction) is the inability to achieve and maintain an erection sufficient to permit satisfactory intercourse.
- It is common, affecting to some extent, 50% of all men over the age of 40 years and the majority of men over 60 years old.
- Most men with impotence suffer in silence and embarrassment. It can lead to great unhappiness and depression and can cause major problems in relationships.
- Many men with coronary heart disease are impotent to some degree. This may be due to their age or the narrowing process in the arteries to the penis.
- Impotence often affects men with angina or those who have had a heart attack, heart surgery, or angioplasty.
- Men or their wives or partners may be worried that sex may be dangerous and cause a heart attack. It rarely does.
- Impotence is more common in men who smoke and who have high blood pressure, diabetes, and high cholesterol. It may be caused by alcohol. Most men with impotence have at least one of these risk factors.
- It may also be caused by several drugs used to treat coronary heart disease and its risk factors. Stopping the drug responsible may cure the impotence.
- It is common in men who are depressed or stressed for any reason, and who do not have coronary heart disease.
- It is also caused by other medical conditions.
- Sex is not dangerous to people who have coronary heart disease, or heart failure, as long as they do not have angina, or severe breathlessness at rest or upon minimal exertion.
- Impotence may improve if it is related to stress or cardiovascular problems that can be improved.
- The new PDE-5 inhibitors, for example, sildenafil (Viagra), are often helpful.

SEX, ANGINA, AND HEART ATTACKS

Is It Dangerous to Have Sex if Patients Have Angina or Have Had a Heart Attack?

Active sex is like other forms of exercise that increase the heart rate and blood pressure. Sex for men without heart problems may cause breathlessness. In men with coronary heart disease, it may cause angina and rarely cause heart attacks. It is difficult to know if, or how often, sex has caused death due to a heart attack because it is difficult to find out and not the sort of question that is volunteered or asked at the time. Although theoretically, vigorous sex can trigger a heart attack (like severe exercise or stress), heart attacks occur for many reasons we do not understand. Most heart attacks do not occur during or shortly after sex.

When Is It Safe to Have Sex after a Heart Attack?

It is probably safe to have sex after a heart attack as soon as the person is able to walk half a mile or up a flight of stairs without angina or breathlessness. The time it takes for people to feel in the mood for sex and self-confident varies a lot, from a few weeks to months. Patients and/or their partners who are scared to have sex because they think it would be dangerous should speak to their internist or cardiologist.

Cardiac rehabilitation courses offer the opportunity to discuss these issues. It is also worthwhile for patients to discuss these things with their doctor or nurse, who should be able to provide advice and reassurance.

CAN IMPOTENCE BE DUE TO THE DRUGS PATIENTS ARE TAKING?

Almost any drug, or just knowing that you have a heart condition that necessitates taking a drug, may cause or contribute to impotence. Some groups of drugs given to either prevent or treat patients with coronary heart disease are particularly likely to cause impotence. These are:

- beta blockers (drugs ending in "–ol"), which are used to treat high blood pressure, angina, and heart failure and are also given to patients after heart attacks

- thiazide diuretics (water tablets, which end in "-ide"), which are used to treat high blood pressure
- statins (drugs ending in "-statin"), which are used to lower a high cholesterol level and are also given to patients with narrowing of the arteries
- angiotensin converting enzyme inhibitors, or "ACE inhibitors" (drugs ending in "-pril"), which are used to treat high blood pressure and coronary or other types of arterial blockages.

ARE ALL DRUGS IN THE GROUP THE SAME, WITH THE SAME SIDE EFFECTS?

Yes, pretty much.

There are several drugs (made by different companies) within each group or family of drugs. They tend to be very similar, with only slight differences, because they have a similar chemical structure. Usually, if one of the group causes impotence, another will do the same. Sometimes, it's worth switching to another drug in the same group to find out. If a drug causes impotence, stopping it should cure the problem. If it doesn't, it is unlikely that the drug is responsible. Patients with impotence should discuss this with their internist or cardiologist.

WHAT SHOULD MEN DO IF ONE OF THEIR HEART TABLETS MAY BE CAUSING IMPOTENCE?

It may not be necessary to stop the drug that may be causing or contributing to their impotence. The doctor may suggest that they continue with the drug and take an extra drug called a PDE-5 inhibitor.

ARE THESE THE VIAGRA TABLETS?

Yes. The new group of drugs, called phosphodiesterase type-5 inhibitors (PDE-5-drugs ending in "tadalafil"), of which sildenafil (or Viagra) was the first, may help. Others (tadalfil, vardenafil) are available. They are safe and useful in most men with impotence. Depending on what other conditions the man has, for example, diabetes, his internist or cardiologist may be able to

13

give him a prescription for it. Beware of getting them on the Internet. It may not be the real thing.

ARE DRUGS LIKE VIAGRA SAFE FOR MEN WITH ANGINA AND WHO HAVE HAD HEART ATTACKS?

Yes, as long as the men do not have angina at rest or during minimal activities. Some men may have had an exercise test. If they did well, and did not get angina or a major abnormality on the recording of their heart (ECG), it would be safe for them to take these drugs.

CAN MEN TAKE ONE OF THESE DRUGS FOR IMPOTENCE IF THEY TAKE DRUGS FOR THEIR HEART?

Because they can lower the blood pressure, PDE-5 tablets are not given to patients who take nitrates (e.g., isosorbide, GTN) in any form for their angina. They are not usually given to patients who have had a recent (less than a month ago) heart attack, heart bypass, stroke or to those who get angina when at rest or when doing very little activity (unstable angina). This is because the PDE-5 tablet may lower the blood pressure and reduce the amount of blood getting to the heart, causing a heart attack.

WHAT ARE THE OTHER SIDE EFFECTS OF THESE TYPES OF DRUGS?

Headache and a red face.

HOW SHOULD THEY BE TAKEN?

Men should take them half an hour before they want to have sex. They take about 30 minutes to work and the effect lasts about 3 to 6 hours. Men should read the instructions on the sheet in the box or speak to the prescribing physician or the pharmacist.

WHEN CAN PATIENTS HAVE SEX AFTER HEART SURGERY OR ANGIOPLASTY?

Impotence is quite common after a heart procedure. Most patients do not ask about sexual matters with their doctor or the nurses in hospital, probably because when they come into the hospital and when recovering from heart surgery, sex is not the most pressing thing on their minds. There are no rules about sex after either coronary artery surgery or angioplasty. Most of it is common sense. No trials have been done about how, where, and when sex can or should be safely resumed after these procedures.

- **Heart bypass surgery**
  The breastbone (sternum) is usually cut (actually with an electric saw!) to allow the surgeon to get at the heart to do the operation. It takes several weeks for the breastbone to knit. Therefore, it is important that it is not displaced or put out of alignment. If it is, it won't heal and it can be very painful and unpleasant. Although it may take around 12 weeks for it to heal completely, it is probably safe to have sex before the 12-week period is over as long as no pressure is put on the breastbone.
  Some heart bypass operations are now done without cutting the breastbone, making a much smaller cut in the side of the ribs (minimally invasive bypass). Sex can resume earlier in these cases.

- **Angioplasty**
  This is less complicated because the procedure involves putting a small tube in the artery in the groin (femoral artery), and patients leave the hospital the following day and can resume all activities around a week later. They could resume sex as soon as their leg has healed and is not sore.

13

Tests and Procedures for Angina and Heart Attacks

Read this chapter to find out about what the commonly performed tests for angina and heart attacks involve.

ELECTROCARDIOGRAM (ECG)

What Is It?

This is a test of the electrical activity of the heart. It is used to diagnose heart attacks in people with chest pain.

It tells us the heart rhythm, the heart rate, if there has been a heart attack or the early signs of a heart attack; whether the passage of electrical messages through the heart is normal—this would be abnormal if the electrical wiring of the heart is faulty. The ECG also provides information on the thickness of the walls of the pumping chamber, which may be affected in patients with high blood pressure or a very narrowed outflow (aortic) valve. Some people have an abnormally thick wall of their pumping chamber (left ventricle), and this uncommon condition (hypertrophic cardiomyopathy) is often picked up when an ECG is done for other reasons, for example, as part of health screening.

When Is an ECG Used?

- **Angina**
  The ECG is usually normal in angina except when the patient has unstable angina with intermittent blocking of the heart artery.

- **Heart attack**
  It will be abnormal and remain abnormal in over 90% of patients who have had a heart attack. A normal ECG in a person with chest pain, unlikely to be due to the heart (for example, indigestion), would exclude a heart attack. The ECG may need to be repeated if it is initially normal in people suspected of having a heart attack, because sometimes the signs of a heart

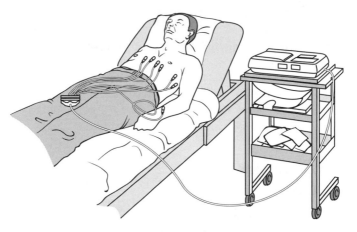

Figure 14.1: Diagram of ECG being recorded.

attack only appear on the ECG after a few hours. Some people with a heart attack may initially have a normal ECG.

- **Palpitations** – awareness of the heartbeat
  If recorded while the patient is having palpitations, the ECG is very useful. It may show an abnormal heart rhythm at the time the patient is feeling the palpitations. It may be normal, showing that the cause of the palpitations is not related to a disturbance of the heart's rhythm.

- **Heart failure**
  A normal ECG makes heart failure unlikely.

How Is an ECG Done?

1. The patient lies quietly and still on a table, having stripped to the waist.
2. In order to get good electrical contact between the electrodes (which detect the heart's electrical activity through the skin) and the skin, the skin may be cleaned with alcohol and rubbed with fine sandpaper. Men may need to have the hair on their chest shaved.
3. Six electrodes are stuck on the chest in certain positions, one on each wrist, and one just above each ankle.
4. These electrodes are connected to the ECG machine with clips attached to cables.
5. It takes less than a minute.

Are There Any Dangers?

None.
It does not hurt.
It is not dangerous to pregnant women.

WHAT IS AN EXERCISE TEST (STRESS TEST)

It is an ECG recorded at rest and also during exercise to see if there is enough blood getting to the heart during exercise.

When Is It Used?

It is used in patients with chest pain or those suspected of having coronary heart disease. The goal of the test is to stress the heart by increasing the heart rate and blood pressure. If the person has normal heart arteries, there will be plenty of blood and oxygen getting to the heart muscle through the heart arteries. The patient should be able to do a reasonable amount of exercise (for example, 10 minutes, without chest pain or undue breathlessness, and there should be no ECG changes).

This is the most commonly performed test for people with chest pain. A test is usually defined as "positive" (suggesting a lack of blood to the heart because at least one of the heart arteries is blocked) on the basis of a change in the ECG recorded while the patient is exercising, or if the patient experiences chest discomfort during exercise.

If the patient does not experience chest discomfort and there are no ECG changes, this "negative" result, in a person who is unlikely to have coronary heart disease, would be very reassuring.

The test is not perfect. This means that some people with coronary heart disease may have a normal "negative" test result ("false negative") while others, who have a normal heart, may have an abnormal test ("false positive") which is common in young women.

The test is most helpful in patients who have an "*intermediate*" risk of coronary heart disease. These are people who fall in between those who are at "*low*" risk of having coronary heart disease (young people with no angina and no risk factors) and those at "*high*" risk or who do have coronary heart disease (those with angina or who have had a heart attack or angioplasty or heart bypass surgery).

14

- **People at low risk where coronary heart disease is very unlikely**

  An abnormal test result in someone who is very unlikely to have coronary heart disease (young people who do not have risk factors and whose symptoms are unlikely to be due to their heart) would be a "false positive" (the result is falsely and incorrectly positive).

  A normal test result (true negative) tells us what we already know; coronary heart disease is very unlikely.

- **People at high risk where coronary heart disease is very likely**

  A normal test result in someone who is very likely to have coronary heart disease (old people with angina and more than one risk factor) would be a "false negative" (a false and incorrect normal or negative result).

  An abnormal result (true positive) tells us what we already know; the person is likely to have coronary heart disease.

How Is It Done?

1. The patient's skin is prepared in the same way as for an ECG (see above).
2. They should wear comfortable shoes and trousers. Women should wear a sports bra.
3. Patients are exercised on a stationary bicycle or a treadmill (similar to the ones in a gym).
4. Their blood pressure is recorded at the beginning and during the test.
5. The ECG is recorded during the test.
6. It is not necessary to stop heart medication before the test.

What Are the Dangers?

The risk of death is 1 in 100,000 and applies mainly to people with badly narrowed heart arteries or those with unstable angina. People at high risk are not usually exercised. Except in people with very bad angina at rest (in whom the test is not necessary and should not be done), the test is safe even in people who have had a recent heart attack, as long as they are not getting angina. A supervised exercise test in the hospital, where patients can be treated and resuscitated if necessary, is safer for them than walking in the street or walking upstairs at home without the safety of a doctor with resuscitation equipment.

Does It Hurt?

The aim of the test is to stress the heart and see if enough blood and oxygen are getting to the heart. Therefore, patients are encouraged to do their best and to exercise as much as they can. Patients should, therefore, feel hot, sweaty, and breathless. Patients with coronary heart disease may get angina. If they do get angina, they are offered a glyceryl trinitrate spray or tablet but, usually, the angina passes in a few minutes. If a patient does get angina, then the test has provided useful information. It is helpful to know how long they were able to exercise before they got angina. If the angina came on within a few minutes, they may need to have a special X-ray of the heart arteries (coronary angiogram).

NUCLEAR HEART TESTS FOR PATIENTS WHO ARE SUSPECTED OF HAVING CORONARY HEART DISEASE

What Is a Nuclear Heart Scan?

It is an injection of a radioactive substance through a vein that is taken up into the heart muscle. Scans of the heart are done immediately and six hours after an exercise test to see if all parts of the heart have an equal amount of radioactivity.

These tests provide similar information as an exercise test. The main reason for doing a nuclear test is if a patient has an abnormal ECG appearance, which would make it difficult to interpret during exercise.

How Is It Done?

The test involves injecting a radioactive chemical into a vein during the exercise test (done on either a bicycle or a treadmill) and then doing a scan of the heart at peak exercise to see if the radioactive material has reached all parts of the heart. Another scan is done a few hours later, by which time all parts of the heart would have recovered and all would have the same amount of radioactive material. If a part of the heart gets less radioactive

14

material than others at peak exercise, but gets the same as the other parts of the heart a few hours later, this suggests that the artery supplying that part of the heart may be narrowed.

ARE THEY USEFUL?

Only in a minority of patients.

The test is expensive, time-consuming (7 hours compared to 20 minutes for an exercise test), and invasive (an injection is necessary) and is no more accurate than an exercise test unless the patient's ECG is abnormal. The dose of radioactive material is not dangerous, but it is more dangerous than nothing at all (an exercise test). People with a normal scan are very unlikely to have a heart attack in the next five years.

STRESS ECHOCARDIOGRAPHY (ULTRASOUND)
What Is It?

It is an ultrasound scan of the heart done before and after exercise or during an injection of a drug through a vein into the bloodstream, to stress the heart (increasing the heart rate and blood pressure).

When Is It Used?

It is used for the same reasons as an exercise test.

How Is It Done?

1. An ultrasound scan of the heart is done first with the patient lying on their left side on a couch. Special ultrasound gel is placed on the skin near the breastbone and under the left breast, and a probe (transducer) is pressed firmly against the skin. The doctor or technician can see the walls of the heart squeezing (contracting) and thickening on a TV screen; this is recorded.
2. The heart is stressed, to increase the heart rate and blood pressure, by either exercising the patient (bicycle or treadmill) or with a drug given through a vein in the hand. The purpose

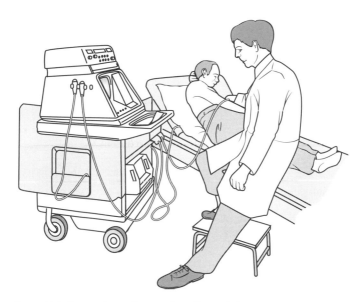

Figure 14.2: Diagram showing how an echocardiogram is done.

of the stress test is to see whether there is enough blood and oxygen getting to the heart when it most needs it.

3. The ultrasound scan is repeated and the pictures at peak stress compared to those at rest.

4. In patients with a normal blood supply to their heart, all sections of the heart muscle walls will squeeze (contract) and thicken more forcibly during exercise. In people with blocked arteries, the wall may not squeeze or thicken as it should. This suggests that the heart muscle wall is not getting enough blood.

5. The wall of the heart in a patient who has had a heart attack may not squeeze or thicken as it should because it is scarred.

6. The wall of the heart in a patient who has not had a heart attack but has a narrowed artery may thicken normally but not squeeze in as fast as it should.

What Are the Drawbacks?

It is time-consuming (around one hour). The person doing it must be good and experienced. Getting good ultrasound pictures

14

of the heart is not possible in all people; they may have a thick or fat chest wall or "overinflated" lungs due to emphysema. Some people feel dizzy and get chest pain when given the drug.

Is It Better or More Accurate Than an Exercise Test?

Slightly, only in people whose ECG makes it difficult to interpret. It is most useful in people with an abnormal ECG.

Is It Dangerous?

Occasionally, the drug used to stress the heart can cause a heart rhythm disturbance, which usually resolves when the infusion is stopped.

ELECTRON BEAM COMPUTED TOMOGRAM (EBCT) OF THE HEART ARTERIES

What Is an EBCT Scan?

It is a CT X-ray scan of the heart arteries looking for calcium in the walls of the arteries. The more calcium in the wall of the artery, the more likely the artery is to be narrowed.

Does It Tell if a Person's Heart Arteries Are Narrowed?

No. The older we get, the more calcium is deposited in the walls of the arteries. So, elderly people would be expected to have more calcium than young people. Some people, particularly elderly people, would be expected to have calcium deposits in the walls of their arteries, but despite this, their arteries may be otherwise normal, without narrowings or blockages. It really tells the age of the arteries, and not whether the arteries are narrowed. Young people may have blobs of fat (atheromatous plaques) in a heart artery but no calcium, and so in both the young and the older patients, the scan may be misleading. The American Heart Association and American College of Cardiology do not recommend these scans for screening purposes.

Does It Predict if Patients Are Going to Have a Heart Attack?

No. There is no evidence that it can detect whether a blob of fat in a heart artery is going to get inflamed, crack, and get blocked off by a blood clot.

Is It Worth Having One Done in Patients Who Have Had a Heart Attack or Blocked Arteries?

No. The scan may be negative and in any case, you already know that you have coronary heart disease.

But if Patients Know They Have Calcium in the Wall of an Artery, Doesn't It Help Them?

No. If their doctor thinks that they have risk factors, they will be advised what to do. The result of the scan would not influence the decision to treat high blood pressure or a high cholesterol level.

Patients who have angina or have had a heart attack will not benefit from an EBCT scan.

Patients who do not have angina or risk factors will not benefit from an EBCT scan.

COMPUTERIZED TOMOGRAPHIC CORONARY ANGIOGRAPHY

This is a new way to do coronary angiography without entering an artery. It is used to tell us if a heart artery is normal or blocked. Because the contrast fluid is injected into a vein and not an artery, the risk of complications is much lower than with arterial angiography.

STRESS MAGNETIC RESONANCE IMAGING

Magnetic resonance imaging does not use X-rays and is safe. It gives better pictures of the heart and arteries than echocardiography.

It is used to see if the heart muscle moves normally during stress (for example, exercise or dobutamine) and at rest. It tells

14

us whether heart muscle is normal or damaged, and also whether there is enough blood getting to the heart muscle.

The test is difficult to do, expensive and not widely available. At the moment, we do not know how useful this test will be.

CORONARY ANGIOGRAM (CARDIAC CATHETER)

What Is It?

It is an X-ray of the heart arteries (angio = artery, gram = picture).

When Is It Done?

To see if the heart (coronary arteries) are narrowed or blocked and how badly. It tells us whether a patient's arteries are normal or not. It is more accurate than any other test.

Coronary angiography is done in patients with angina and those who have had a heart attack. It is also now available in some hospitals at the time a patient is having a heart attack so that angioplasty (opening the artery with a balloon) can be performed (see below).

How Is It Done?

It is done as an outpatient procedure and takes around 30 minutes. Angioplasty done immediately following the angiogram takes an additional 30 to 60 minutes.

Patients should not have eaten or had anything to drink for 4 hours before the procedure although they should take their medication as usual. They should not take the blood thinner (anticoagulant) warfarin for four days before because they might get prolonged bleeding and a big bruise and lump (hematoma) over the skin. Diabetics taking a drug called metformin should not take it for 24 hours either before or after the angiogram because it can interact with the contrast fluid, causing kidney damage.

1. The procedure and the risks are explained, and the patient signs a consent form. The area at the top of the right leg (groin) is shaved so that hair does not get into the skin, causing infection. Patients wear only a gown.

2. Patients (if they are able) walk into the X-ray room (cardiac catheter laboratory) and lie on a narrow, hard table. A large cylinder (the X-ray equipment) is placed near their chest. ECG electrodes are put on the chest, hands, and feet.

3. In the "cath lab," there are one or two nurses, a technician to record and monitor the heart rate and the pressures within the heart measured by the catheter (tube) placed into the artery at the top of the leg (femoral artery), and a radiographer responsible for taking pictures of the heart arteries. The cardiologist scrubs (washes the hands and arms) and puts on a gown and gloves.

4. Sedation may be given to patients who want it or who are very nervous.

5. The patients' shaved groin (usually the right) is then washed with antiseptic fluid, which can sting. The patient is covered, neck to feet, with a paper drape. The patient should lie still and keep their hands by their sides so as not to desterilize the groin area.

6. Local anesthetic is then injected into the skin and tissues over the groin (femoral) artery; this can sting.

7. A needle is inserted into the groin artery (which should not hurt). A short tube (sheath) with a valve to prevent blood flowing out is then put into the groin artery. Catheters are then threaded through the sheath and positioned in the heart arteries. This is done by using the X-ray to see where the tubes are. There are two heart arteries (the left and the right coronary arteries). Differently shaped catheters, specially shaped to fit into each coronary artery, are inserted separately into each artery. Contrast fluid is injected into each artery while taking X-ray pictures. The X-ray tube moves around to take pictures of the arteries from different positions. Several pictures are taken of each artery in different projections and angles, to make sure that what appears to be a narrowing really is a narrowing rather than a bend in the artery.

8. Pictures are taken of the left heart pumping chamber (left ventricle) using a separate catheter. The injection of contrast fluid into the pumping chamber often causes a flushing feeling, and some patients feel that they have urinated and should be warned about this before the injection. The flushed feeling lasts less than 10 seconds and is not unpleasant.

14

---

9. The tube is removed from the artery, and the artery is then pressed for a few minutes to stop the bleeding, or a special plug is inserted through a tube to seal the hole in the artery. This allows the patient to get out of bed earlier.

10. Patients are then asked to lie flat for at least an hour or two to make sure that there is no bleeding from the groin artery. They then sit up for a little while and can go home. They are encouraged to drink and can eat immediately after the test.

11. Patients are not allowed to drive home. It is preferred that they are driven home rather than use public transport. They should not go to work that day but can go back to work on the following day assuming they feel well and the groin has healed.

12. Most cardiologists tell the patient the result and explain what needs to be done (if anything) before the patient leaves the hospital.

13. If the arteries are normal, this is very good news and means that the patient does not need medication for their heart although they may need other tablets, for example, for a high cholesterol level or high blood pressure. Patients with slight narrowing of the arteries should take aspirin.

14. Patients with important narrowings may be advised to have ballooning (coronary angioplasty) of one or more arteries, or coronary artery bypass grafting, or if a valve is not working properly, valve surgery. These are sometimes difficult decisions, and the patient may be referred to a different consultant or heart surgeon.

What Are the Risks?

- Occasionally, less than 1 in 100 cases, but particularly in the elderly and those with high blood pressure or a leaky outflow (aortic) heart valve, there may be an aneurysm in the groin artery. This gets bigger and more painful over a few days after the angiogram, and this needs urgent treatment. Patients should contact and see the cardiologist so that the aneurysm can be treated. Sometimes a small operation is necessary.

- Most patients have some, usually slight, bruising over the artery, which settles down over a few days.

- The risk of death, a heart attack, or a stroke is 1 in 1000, but this is mainly in the elderly and those with very bad arteries.
- One in 100 patients gets a red rash over the body as a reaction to the contrast fluid. This usually goes away on its own within a day or two. Patients who get a rash should call the hospital or see their doctor so that it can go on their record in case they have another, similar procedure in the future.

CORONARY ANGIOPLASTY

What Is It?

This is a commonly used procedure, not a test, to treat patients with blocked or narrowed arteries, who may have angina or have had a heart attack. The procedure is similar to a coronary angiogram and often follows immediately after a coronary angiogram. It is used to treat patients very soon after they have had a heart attack, as soon as they come into the hospital.

It involves widening a narrowed artery, or unblocking a blocked artery, by passing a very thin wire down the heart artery and then, threaded on top of this wire, using a special tube with a small plastic balloon at the end to widen the artery. All of this is done from the groin artery; the movement and positioning of the wire and the balloon are done using X-rays. The procedure can often be completed within half an hour, although complicated cases can take longer.

Stainless steel meshwork cylinders averaging 3 mm in diameter are usually put in the artery during the procedure to reduce the risk of the artery blocking off soon after the procedure and the stent also reduces the risk of the artery narrowing down again later.

Angioplasty (widening of an artery) is also used to widen narrowed arteries in the neck (carotid) arteries, the kidney (renal) artery, and the leg arteries.

Before the Procedure

Patients should not eat or drink for four hours before the procedure, but should take all their medication with a glass of water

14

on the day of the procedure. Diabetics should not take their metformin for one day before and one day after the procedure because the combination of contrast fluid and metformin can cause kidney damage. Stopping metformin for a couple of days is not dangerous.

The procedure and the risks and benefits are explained to the patient (and their family) if they wish. This should be done in a clinic as well as when patients are admitted to the hospital. If patients are in any doubt or wish to change their mind about having the procedure, the procedure may be cancelled or postponed.

WHAT ARE THE RISKS OF ANGIOPLASTY?

There is a 2% risk of heart attack, stroke, death or need for urgent heart bypass surgery.

Angioplasty, like any procedure, should not be done if the risks of the procedure are greater than the risks of not having it done.

Because a tube is placed in the groin artery and because heparin is given, most patients will get a bruise in the groin. Around 2% of patients may get a big blood lump (hematoma) in the groin, which usually settles down with bruising spreading down the leg, over a week or two. It is best to rest the leg and avoid vigorous walking and exercise until it settles down. If it doesn't get better, or if it gets worse, patients should see their doctor.

Less commonly, particularly in the elderly and patients with high blood pressure, who have hard, chalky arteries, there may be a "blow out" or false aneurysm in the wall of the artery. This may be painful and cause throbbing and swelling where the tube was inserted in the groin artery. The patient should contact the cardiologist and should be seen immediately for an examination. An ultrasound scan will show if there is a problem, the size of the communication between the artery and the blow out sac (false aneurysm) in the wall of the artery (like a blow out in a car tyre). If small, it may get better on its own. If big, a clotting medicine (thrombin) can be injected into the sac, using the ultrasound scanner to help locate the sac. Once the sac is closed, the communication is closed and the problem heals over a few weeks.

THE ANGIOPLASTY PROCEDURE

1. The procedure is performed in the cardiac X-ray room (cardiac catheter laboratory). The patient lies on a rather firm X-ray table. Some patients like a small dose of sedative (Valium) given as an injection.

2. The patient's groin (usually the right) is washed and a large paper drape is placed over the patient, leaving only a small hole over the groin area. Local anesthetic, which stings a bit, like a bee sting, is then injected into the skin. A needle is then put through the skin into the artery (femoral) just below the groin crease.

3. A very thin, soft steel wire is then threaded through the needle into the artery. The needle is removed and a plastic tube (called a "sheath") is then threaded over the wire and left in the artery, and the wire removed. The tube has a valve that allows other tubes to be threaded through it but does not allow blood to flow out. Heparin, a medicine to stop blood clotting in the tubes and the arteries, is given in a dose that is sufficient to prevent blood clots, but not too much to cause excessive bleeding. The patient's blood stickiness is measured during the procedure. Where possible, other drugs, including aspirin and drugs like aspirin, are given before the procedure to reduce the risk of blood clotting in the first few days or weeks after the procedure. All these drugs can lead to bleeding, which increases the risks of bleeding in the groin and occasionally elsewhere.

4. A long, fairly stiff plastic tube (called a catheter) is then threaded, under X-ray control, to the heart artery where the problem is. The catheters come in various shapes and sizes, designed to fit safely and firmly in the heart artery. There are several differently shaped catheters for each artery depending on the shape and size of the patient. Pictures of the arteries are taken to make sure that the catheter is stable and is firmly seated in the mouth of the heart artery, and also to check the site and appearance of the narrowing.

14

5. A very thin wire (called a guidewire) is then threaded, under X-ray control, through the catheter, and down the heart artery. The end of the guidewire in the heart can be turned in all directions by small gentle twists at the other end, which is jutting outside the sheath. The guidewire is pushed gently down the artery, through the narrowing or the blockage. Different types and strengths or hardness of guidewires are selected, depending on whether the artery is blocked or just narrowed.
6. With the wire held in position down the narrowed artery, the balloon catheter [a long, thin, flexible, hollow plastic tube with a deflated balloon and stainless steel cage (or stent) attached firmly over the balloon] is then threaded over the guidewire. The balloon has steel markers on it, and so the balloon can be positioned at the narrowed part of the artery, using the X-ray machine. When the operator is satisfied that the balloon and the stent are in the correct position, the balloon is inflated using a special syringe attached to its other end.
7. The balloon is filled with contrast fluid, so that the full balloon with the expanded stent can be seen with the X-ray. The balloon expands, opening up the stent and squashing the fatty material (atheroma) in the artery against the walls. As the balloon is inflated, the stent is pressed against the walls of the artery. The steel mesh of the stent can be seen on the X-ray. The steel mesh acts as scaffolding and prevents any tears or rips in the wall of the artery falling back into the artery, causing a blockage. Once expanded, the stent does not collapse. The stent holds the torn bits of the artery back against the wall.
8. After the stent has been fully expanded (by fully inflating the balloon), the balloon is then deflated by sucking the contrast back into the syringe. The stent remains expanded. The balloon catheter is then pulled back. The wire is sometimes pulled back with the balloon but is sometimes left in the artery while check pictures are taken to make sure that no further treatments are necessary at other sites in the artery.

Today's stents are coated with drugs that also reduce the chance that the artery will narrow down (restenosis). Restenosis used to occur in 30% of cases before we had stents. The stainless steel stents arrived in the early 1990s and reduced the risk of restenosis from 30% to 10%. With the new coated stents, restenosis occurs in around 2% of cases.

WHAT CAN GO WRONG?

- All the things that can go wrong with a coronary angiogram.
- Clots can occasionally (4% of cases) form in the stent because it acts as a "foreign body" in the artery, with blood clotting cells (platelets) sticking to it.
- The artery can tear and block off, causing a heart attack (1%) or death. The risks depend on several factors: the age of the patient, whether he or she has had a recent heart attack, the strength of the heart muscle, the number of arteries affected, whether the patient has diabetes, whether the patient smokes or has high blood pressure and other risk factors.

14

About the Authors

Dr. Clive Handler, BSc, MD, MRCP, FACC, FESC, is Consultant in the National Pulmonary Hypertension Unit at The Royal Free Hospital, London; Honorary Senior Lecturer in the Department of Medicine, The Royal Free and University College Medical School, London; and Consultant Cardiologist at Highgate Hospital, London. He was previously Consultant Cardiologist at Northwick Park and St Mary's Hospitals, London. He trained at Guy's Hospital Medical School and at St Luke's Hospital, Milwaukee, University of Wisconsin. His textbook *Cardiology in Primary Care* was published by Radcliffe Publishing in 2004. He co-edited *Classic Papers in Coronary Angioplasty* with Dr. Michael Cleman from Yale University Medical School (Springer) and edited *Guy's Hospital – 250 years* in 1975. His forthcoming books include *Prevention of Cardiovascular Disease in Primary Care* and *Management of Cardiac Problems in Primary Care* (both written with Dr. Gerry Coghlan and published by Radcliffe Publishing) and is co-editor of *Vascular Complications in Human Disease: Mechanisms and Consequences* (Springer). He has written numerous scientific papers.

Dr. Gerry Coghlan, MD, FRCP, is Consultant Cardiologist and Director of the National Pulmonary Hypertension Unit at the Royal Free Hospital. He trained in Dublin and at Harefield and the Royal Free Hospitals. He is an international authority on Pulmonary Hypertension but has wide interests in all aspects of the management of coronary heart disease and angioplasty. He has written several books with Dr. Clive Handler as well as scientific papers on pulmonary hypertension and other aspects of cardiology.

Index

Antidepressants, 201
    alcohol and, 138
    tricyclic, 201
Antioxidants, 119
Anxiety, 56, 195; *see also* Stress
    after heart attack, 101
    management, 200–201
    traits, 201
Aorta, 24, 33, 55–56
    aneurysm, 17, 33–34
    dissection of, 17, 56
    narrowing, 17, 164
Aortic regurgitation, 26
Aortic stenosis, 25–26
    problems due to, 26, 51
Aortic valve, 24
    problems, 25–26, 51
Appraisals, work, 198
Arteries, 12, 21, 22, 34; *see also*
                Arterioles; Capillaries
    definition, 33
Arterioles, 32, 34, 160
Aspirin, 16, 68
    after angioplasty, 243
    after heart attack, 95, 100, 108
    after heart bypass surgery, 80
    complications, 106
    diabetic patients and, 106, 155
    in women, 219
Atenolol, 166, 194
Atheroma, 1, 50, 120, 132, 208
Atherosclerosis, 1–2
    sites, 18, 121
    stages, 9–10, 120
Athlete's heart, 31
Atria, 24
Atrial fibrillation, 91, 191
Atrioventricular node, 40

B

Balloon catheter, 244
Bendrofluazide, 166
Beta blockers, 16, 68–69, 166, 194
    after heart attack, 71, 96, 100
    side effects, 69, 166, 224
Biguanides, 153
Bile acid sequestrants, 127
Birth control pill, *see* Oral
                contraceptive pill

Blindness, 154
Blood clots, 35, 108
Blood pressure, 32
    checking, 60, 161
        at home, 165
    control, 160–161
    diastolic, 21, 163
    high, *see* Hypertension
    ideal, 162–163
    low, 163–164
    measurement units, 32
    "super low", 154–155
    systolic, 21, 162, 163
    variation in, 37, 161
Blood sugar, high, effects, 153–154
Blood tests, 60
Body mass index (BMI), 130
Brachial artery, 33
Bradycardia, 37–38
Breast cancer, 208, 217
Breathlessness, 26; *see also*
                Emphysema
    angina and, 47
    smoking and, 37
Bronchi, 36
Bronchitis, 28
    and heart failure, 31
Bundle branch block, 65
Bupropion, 176

C

Calcium
    in artery walls, 236, 237
    need for, 70
Calcium channel blockers, 70, 166,
        219
Calories, 131
    content in foods, 134–135
Cancer
    as cause of death, 14–15
    effects of exercise, 141
    smoking and, 172
Cannula, 93
Capillaries, 34
Carbon monoxide, 172
Cardiac arrest, 90
    asystolic, 91
    prognosis, 93
    tests after, 93

---

from peer pressure, 185
from personal problems, 183–184
prevention, 202, 204–205
reducing
   by helping others, 195
   lifestyle changes, 192–193
   steps in, 191–192
   through laughter and humor,
     195–196
severe, 179
   as heart attack trigger, 197
sleep and, 191, 193
social support in combating,
   185–186
start of, 186
stimulation vs, 178
sunshine benefits on, 190
symptoms of syndrome, 180
teaching children about, 199
travel, 189
in women, *see* Women, stress in
Stress echocardiography, *see*
   Echocardiography
Stress testing, *see* Exercise testing
Strokes, 17
Sugar, minimization in diet, 133
Sulphonyureas, 153
Super-foods, 102, 133
Sympathetic nervous system, 40
Syncope (fainting), 26, 161, 164
Syndrome X, 50
Systole, 21, 22, 162

T

Tablets, nicotine, 176
Tachycardia, 38
Tar, 172
Temporal artery, 33
Thiazide, 225
Thrombin, 242
Thrombolytics, 72, 95
Thrombosis, exercise and risk of, 141
Transient ischaemic attack, 124
Tricuspid valve, 24–25
   problems, 27–28
Triglycerides, 117, 156
   level reduction, 126, 127
Troponin, 94–95, 98
"Type A" personality, 196

U

Ulcers
   duodenal, 53
   stomach, 53
Unstable plaques, 50, 120

V

Valium, 243
Valves, *see also* Aortic valve; Mitral
     valve; Pulmonary valve;
     Tricuspid valve
   problems with, 25–29
   and heart failure, 31
Vardenafil, 225
Varicose veins, 35–36
Vasodilators, 32
Veins, 34, 35
   cholesterol not in, 17–18
Ventricles, 24
   left, 24
   right, 25
Ventricular fibrillation, 12, 48, 91, 92
Ventricular septum, 24, 105
Verapamil, 70
VF arrest, *see* Ventricular fibrillation
Viagra, 70, 225–226
Vitamins, 131, 133
   B12, 34
   E, 119–120

W

Warfarin, 138, 238
Water tablets, 166
   thiazide, 225
Weight, ways of losing, 116, 136
"White coat syndrome", 162
Wine, red, and heart disease risk, 136,
   138
Women
   aspirin taking by, 219
   coronary angioplasty in, 220
   coronary artery surgery in, 220
   diabetes in, 213
   heart problems in, 207–221
     angina symptoms, 213,
      215–216
     diagnosis, 211–212, 215–216
     heart attack symptoms,
      214–215, 216